D0429371

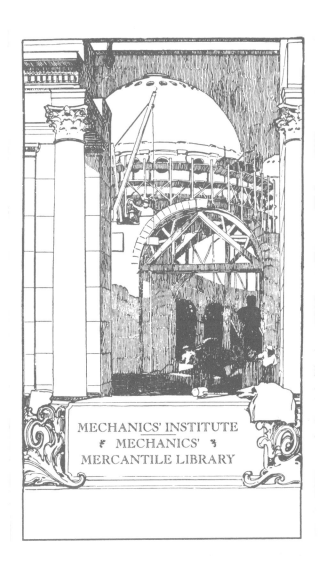

MECHANICS' INSTITUTE
⚜ MECHANICS' ⚜
MERCANTILE LIBRARY

MECHANICS' INSTITUTE

Qigong

Qigong

Chinese Medicine or Pseudoscience?

Lin Zixin, Yu Li, Guo Zhengyi,
Shen Zhenyu, Zhang Honglin,
and Zhang Tongling

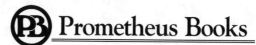 Prometheus Books

59 John Glenn Drive
Amherst, New York 14228-2197

Published 2000 by Prometheus Books

Inquiries should be addressed to
Prometheus Books, 59 John Glenn Drive, Amherst, New York 14228–2197.
VOICE: 716–691–0133, ext. 207.
FAX: 716–564–2711.
WWW.PROMETHEUSBOOKS.COM

04 03 02 01 00   5 4 3 2 1

Library of Congress Cataloging-in-Publication Data

Qigong : Chinese medicine or pseudoscience / Lin Zixin ... [et al.].
      p.   cm.
   ISBN 1–57392–232–3 (cloth : alk. paper)
   1. Ch'i kung. 2. Medicine, Chinese. I. Lin, Zixin.
RA781.8.Q54   1999
615.5'3—dc21   99–36666
                                                                                         CIP

Printed in the United States of America on acid-free paper

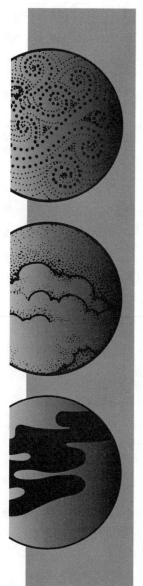

Contents

Preface

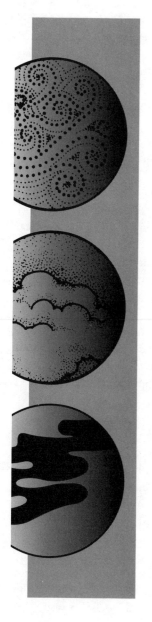

As we look back at human history, we see that various peoples and nations throughout the world created distinctive civilizations. Some of these civilizations continued, some failed to progress, some were drowned out, while others persevered though their progress was labored on their historical path to the present day. That the Chinese nation, with an uninterrupted civilized culture of more than 5,000 years, could be passed down successfully to this day is worth exploring; perhaps that is why this Oriental civilization attracts so much attention in our modern scientific world of interaction and interdependence.

There are many reasons for a nation to continue and progress, rather than disappearing under the pressure of natural catastrophe and man-made calamities. One of the major prerequisites may be its health care and disease-prevention activities. The art of medical treatment and health preservation is one significant aspect of the characteristic Chinese culture. Because cultural exchange among the peoples of the world had not been extensive, there emerged a sense of mystery surrounding Chinese culture. Apart from certain philosophical ideas, the core of this mysticism concerned the art of medical treatment and preserving people's health. In the 1970s the art of acupuncture and moxibustion swept across the globe, and the ranks of kung fu (martial arts) followers have been growing ever since. By the 1980s, the popularity of Chinese Qigong began to grow rapidly, stirring up intense excitement not only in its homeland, but also beyond China's boundaries.

The art of acupuncture and moxibustion were generally accepted by the people of the world because they could allegedly achieve predictable physiological effects. Though we do not fully understand its physiological mechanism, we are sure we will find the answer to this enigma through scientific investigation. But the spread of Qigong has been different from that of acupuncture and moxibustion. Over the last few years the Qigong craze has gotten out of hand, and a lot of puzzling aberrations have occurred in both its promotion and practice. Qigong thus suffers greatly due to ignorance, backwardness, pseudoscience, and antiscience. Meanwhile, due to the appearance of many implausible conclusions that resulted from either popular demonstrations or mistaken public opinions, an increasing number of people began to feel disappointed, skeptical, and befuddled.

Qigong is a part of the cultural heritage of the Chinese nation. It can be practiced without the aid of drugs anywhere one likes, and, when mastered, will serve to balance one's vitality, supplement one's energy, stamp out disease, and promote one's health. But we must point out as well that practice without appropriate training may lead one to "lose control and bring in demoniacness," to use Chinese terminology, or to "induce psychosis," to use modern medical terminology. This is absolutely what we must avoid. In recent years, plenty of charlatans emerged throughout China. They created a lot of publicity for themselves, pretending to be Qigong masters by resorting to all sorts of conjuring tricks, cheating, and pseudoscience. It not only created considerable confusion within China, but also perplexed the outside world. For this reason, we invited experts in this field to write this book in an attempt to promote some thoroughgoing reform.

In this book we will present the origin and historical development of Qigong. Qigong had been, in fact, proceeding along the same lines as witchcraft, but later isolated itself and headed in a different direction. Today's depraved sects of Qigong are by no means the true representation of Qigong. They represent only the return to witchcraft.

We are going to expose the tricks of these charlatans to let more people see the truth and make a correct judgment. At the same time, we must remind the readers that, due both to the influence of certain ideas and to popular scientific illiteracy, the false and the fake may now and then overtake the real–just like the case of the alleged psychic Israeli-born Uri Geller, who is believed by many to have deceived not only the public, but scientists as well.

We are also going to expose some so-called scientific experiments. Cheating in the scientific field is not uncommon; however, such cheating could hardly withstand proper scientific examination, because it cannot be verified unconditionally. So a faked experiment can never be scientific. It is similar to demonstrations of parapsychology, which have been disputed for ages; but here it appears with distinctively Chinese characteristics.

As regards the "emission of energy power" (discharging vital energy to other persons through Qigong exercises to cure disease) and "energy power-dominated lectures" (a variety of so-called energy emission lectures given to large audiences under the control of energy power, usually through the subtle directions by the lecturer), we have also put forth our own distinct opinions. In some countries there are psychotherapies whose origin can be traced back to the primitive practices of witchcraft healing activities. Maybe the phrase "faith makes effect" illustrates the basis of psychotherapeutics, and it is true also in China. As for the effect of the emission of energy power, we believe it has nothing to do with energy power, but is exactly the same as the passionate response of an enthusiastic audience excited by the performances of rock stars. This has already been proved in China in actual instances.

China has an old saying that "domestic shame should not be made public." But we believe we should maintain a respectful attitude toward science, truth, and facts, rather than hide the facts. In compiling this book we aim not to deny our culture, but to allow the people of the world to have a bona fide comprehension of what Qigong is, to better enable them to distinguish the true from the false, and to join together with them in a scientific attitude to illuminate this treasure of scientific culture that belongs to all humankind.

Please note: The authors of this book present examples of Qigong to illustrate their argument. **The reader is strongly encouraged not to try these techniques or tricks.**

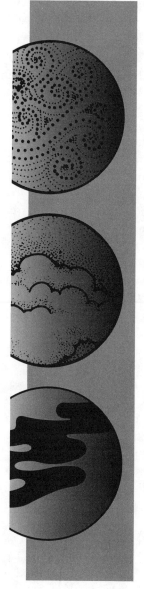

1

Traditional Chinese Medicine and Qigong

Qigong and Its History

Qigong is a personal exercise, a personal form of cultivation, and a personal way of maintaining health. Its history is long and its origin remote. In ancient China the precursors of Qigong were called "Dao Yin," "Tu Na," "Xing Chi," "Tsun Shen," "Hsiu Shen," "Yang Xing," and other names as well. These traditions gradually combined with ancient Chinese philosophy to produce the ancient Qigong methods of strengthening health, a recognized part of traditional Chinese medicine.

From a modern point of view, Qigong is a worthwhile and complete method of exercise. It is a way of controlling and directing the power within a person. The study of Qigong is an anthropological investigation into how to realize human psychological and behavioral control. It falls into the scope of the natural sciences and is closely related to modern preventive medicine, rehabilitative therapy, clinical medicine, geriatrics, sports medicine, psychosomatic medicine, and social medicine. But the applications of Qigong are many: from preventive medicine to various aspects like education, sports, cultural art, military affairs, WuShu (self-defense), aviation, astronavigation training in special or secret careers, or enhancing the potential of human beings.

Historically there have been various schools of Qigong: Yi (medical), Ru (Confucian), Dao (Taoist), Shih (Buddhist), Wu (martial art), Yi (artistic), and others; but in practice they all espouse three principles: regulating the body by practicing forms; regulating the breath and adjusting energy; and regulating the mind and adjusting thought.

Regulating the body is the conscious and deliberate manipulation of the body by holding a set posture for a period of time or performing a set series of movements in order to stimulate the vital parts of the body. *Regulating the breath* is a conscious manipulation of the act of breathing in order to control mental composure and physical condition. Regulating the mind is a conscious effort to control mental activity in order to maintain the mind and body in peak condition. Actually, these are the only three options people have if they wish to regulate their own physical or mental condition. These three principles form the basis of Qigong. That Qigong or its practice is the basis for any discipline in improving one's personal condition is therefore a given.

Qigong developed from ancient medical practices. Of course, it was not the same in antiquity as today's organized Qigong. For example, a person experiencing discomfort in a part of his body will seek relief in massage, manipulation, numbing, or hot or cold therapy to deaden or relieve the pain. One who is tired may yawn or stretch or close one's eyes and keep still for a short time to refresh oneself. One who is under stress or depressed will usually feel better by breathing deeply and exhaling slowly, or by singing out loud, or perhaps by screaming. It is from such simple everyday experiences that Qigong exercises are derived.

The earliest record of Chinese medicine, *The Yellow Emperor's Internal Classic*, refers to and describes ancient types of Qigong. Hsing Chi, Dao Yin, Shou Shen, and others all arose from ancient practices associated with keeping fit. Down to the present, Qigong has been divided into "movement" and "motionless" aspects of exercises. Various literary examples illustrate that Qigong arose from ancient dancelike imitations of the movements of animals, which evolved into imitative Qigong. Such exercises as "turtle flow energy" and "snake flow energy," "dance of the five animals," and others are still practiced today.

In 1957, in the Yueh Du district of Qinghai Province, a clay pot of the MaJia pottery culture was discovered with human figures depicted in postures of the Tu Na school of Qigong (figure 1). This proves that Chinese Qigong's history stretches back at least five thousand years. Many other references to Qigong can be found in pre-Qin dynasty writings, which date before 221 B.C.E.* *The Yellow Emperor's Internal Classic* also mentions Qigong. References to Qigong theory or practice can also be found in the writings of Lao Tse, Zhuang Zi, Confucius, Mencius, and many others, which make clear that Qigong had already passed its rudimentary stages and has become an established discipline. In a literary artifact from the Warring States Period (841–221 B.C.E.) we find the earliest known recorded description of the Tu Na method and philosophy in its complete form. This artifact, known as the "circulating Qi (Energy) jade work," consists of forty-five Chinese characters carved on a small twelve-sided jade post (figure 2).

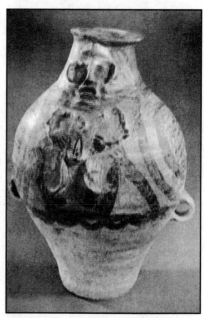

Fig. 1. Clay pot of the MaJia pottery culture with human figures in postures of the Tu Na school of Qigong.

Qigong practices had already become formulated and standardized by the time of the Han dynasty (250 B.C.E.– 220 C.E.). Indeed, the *Dao Yin Illustration* (figure 3), a colored illustration on silk discovered in 1973 at the Ma Wang Burial Site in Chang Sha, Hunan Province demonstrates this; as does the silk scroll called "Fast While Regulating the Breath."

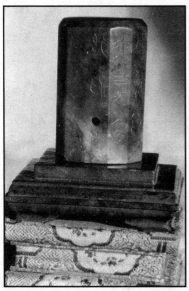

Fig. 2. The circulating Qi jade work is the earliest known recorded description of the Tu Na method.

Zhang Zhong Jing, a famous physician of the Eastern Han dynasty who established the differentiation and treatment system of traditional Chinese medicine, considered Qigong an excellent preventive and therapeutic method, superior to massage or acupuncture. And in the late Han dynasty, Dr. Shen Hua Tuo wrote a description of ancient animal-imitation postures, which he called "Dance of the Five Animals." He recommended this dance for exercising the back and joints and to promote blood and energy circulation. This is not only useful for curing disease, but also an excellent method for preventing disease. The Taoist scholar Wei Bo Yang,★ who in later years was called the Master of the Ancient Dan Writings, defined the basis for the rise of the Nei Dan school of Qigong in the Late Sung dynasty. The physician and Taoist scholar Ge Hong wrote in *Bao Pu Zi* that Tu Na breathing exercises could, by "circulating energy," extend life; and that bending and stretching exercises (Dao Yin) could prevent aging. *Yang Xing Yan Ming Lei* (*Nourish Your Natural State and Extend Your Life*), edited by Tao Hong Jing, was the first literary work that dealt exclusively with Qigong as a means of promoting health.

During the Sui and Tang dynasties and the transient Five-generation period (589–960 C.E.) the court medical personnel included specialists who taught Qigong methods as a means of curing certain diseases in addition to massage and bone adjustment. A high court physician of the Sui dynasty, Chao Yuan Fang, compiled the *Treatise on Etiology and Manifestations of Diseases*, which describes clinical descriptions of various diseases and prescribes only various physical therapies as cures. About two hundred

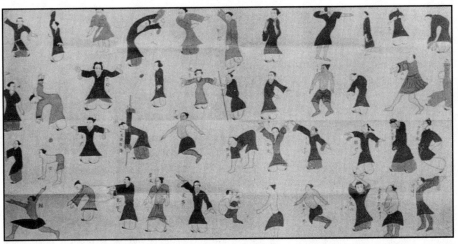

Fig. 3. The *Dao Yin Illustration* shows that Qigong practices had become formulated and standardized by the time of the Han dynasty.

entries are given for Qigong therapies. This book is an extremely valuable research and reference source.

Sun Si Miao, a preeminent specialist in medicine of the Tang dynasty who was familiar with Confucian, Buddhist, and Taoist thought, wrote *Qian Jin Yao Fang (Prescriptions Worth Thousand Gold)* and *Qian Jin Yi Fang (Supplement to Prescriptions Worth Thousand Gold)*. In these books he offered complete advice on nurturing the essential forces of life, and on enunciating Qigong as a regimen for healthy living in systematic form. Dr. Sun himself was a good example of health; he lived past one hundred years and has been honored by later generations with the name Sun Zhen Ren ("Immortal" Sun). These accomplishments illustrate the progress and development of Qigong science, though they still carry some traces of shamanism and animistic superstition.

The Taoist Nei Dan school arose during the Sung and Yuan dynasties (960 C.E.–1367 C.E.), and this greatly influenced Chinese medicine. The Northern Sung emperor commissioned some books. The first of these was *Sheng Ji Zong Lu (Complete Records of the Gathering of Sages)*; this was followed by *Dao Zang (Taoist Scriptures)*, *Shen Xian Dao Yin (Active Qigong Exercise of the Immortals)*, *Shen Xian Fu Qi (Immortals' Breath Control)*, and gion and medicine also had overtones of superstition, and this is quite understandable.

Also during this time the Quan Zhen (Complete Authentic) school of Taoist disciples advocated the methods of quiet cultivation of body and mind and resurrected Lao Tse's *Tao Te Jing* (Dao De Jing) as a canon of instruction. The Complete Authentic School excluded other Taoist beliefs and practices such as the burning of incense and the bowing prayer to spirits and ghosts, astrology and reading mystic signs, the casting of spells, the reciting of incantations, and other superstitious practices.

During the Ming and Ching dynasties (1386–1911) Qigong was used ever more widely in medical applications. Li Shi Zhen, a doctor of medicine, thought the reflective inner examination of the Nei Dan method could give insight into the inner workings of internal organs. The famous doctor Zhang Jing Yue, in a book called *Lei Jing* (*Classification to Internal Classic*), refers many times to the *Dan Scriptures* and expresses the belief that steadfastly practicing Qigong several times a day over a long period of time will result in a fit and healthy body, clear senses, and the prevention of disease.

Dr. Li Yan, in *Yi Xue Ru Men Bao Yang Shuo* (*Introduction to Medicine: A Discussion of Health Care*), criticized Taoist concepts such as "stopping death," "spiritual levitation," and other forms of sorcery, and argued that it is absurd to pursue immortality as if it is not evident that a person's life expectancy is not one hundred years or so at most. To sit with one's eyes closed all day meditating is just a selfish preoccupation; it is not easy to achieve real peace that way. But if one understands the natural rhythms of life, things will be in order naturally; and if one is not greedy or restless or having wild dreams, then the spirit will be happy and the mind at peace; one will achieve peace without effort. Only in this way will one be able to prevent disease, stay healthy, and live to a natural old age. Gao Lian, in *Zun Sheng Ba Jian* (*Eight Commentaries on How to Follow the Law of Life*) wrote, "My life is in my hands; it is not decided by heaven. If I use it without conscience, it will end. If I use it wisely, for good, it will continue." He also wrote, "The way of fetal breath is the source of all the methods of Taoist practice. Dao Yin, therefore, is an important art of Qi-propagation. People can cultivate Qi to preserve their spirit; if Qi (energy) is clear then the spirit will be refreshed. Exercise the body to rid it of disease; the body will live and the disease will leave." Tsao Tsi Shan (Cao

Cishan), in *Lao Lao Heng Yan* (*The Ever-True Old Sayings*), had no interest in Taoism, denying the Taoist ideas of desirelessness, unawareness, propagating Qi through "passes," and internal alchemy. He thought that it is not the way of life-cultivation that the heart be like withered trees or ashes, rather a person should make good use of the heart (mind) but only at peace, for a peaceful spirit results in no exhaustion.

Wang Ang spoke of channeling thought and calming the spirit. In his *Wu Yao Yuan Quan* (*Explanation of the Theory of Do Medicine*) he wrote of the methods of breath regulation and the Minor Celestial Cycle Practice. Shen Jinao, in *Za Beng Yuan Liu Xi Zhu* (*Origin and Progression of Various Diseases*) lists Qigong as a therapy for forty diseases. This is a valuable literary work for selecting Qigong methods in terms of differentiation. In *Nei Gong Tu Shuo* (*Illustrated Explanation of Internal Qigong*), edited by Pan Wei, illustrations were used to explain active and relaxation Qigong exercises in a simple step-by-step detail that laymen could readily understand.

As to recent developments, it is quite apparent that Qigong is enjoying a renaissance thanks to modern science. Although truth is often difficult to uncover, today's methods can slowly improve upon yesterday's traditions.

Basic Methods and Important Facts About Qigong

Throughout its history Qigong has had many schools and groups, each with its own characteristics. Students have had a hard time deciding which group to follow. For this reason, it is necessary to describe Qigong's basic methods and common points. I earlier made reference to the Three Principles; and the practice of Qigong from ancient times to the present, in China and abroad, and by whatever name or method, must begin with the practice of these Three Principles:

1. regulate one's body;
2. regulate one's breath;
3. regulate one's mind.

Some people call these principles the basic methods of Qigong; others call them the secrets of Qigong or the essence of Qigong; and there are other names. No school of Qigong, be it simple or complex in its teachings, strays from these parameters; the various schools differ only in their emphasis on one aspect or the other.

Regulate the body by movement

The most concise explanation of this principle can be given in four words: *movement, stillness, relaxation,* and *tension.* These words can also be applied to the exercises of regulating breath to control Qi (energy) and regulating the mind to control thought. Applying complete concentration to the task of holding a posture can aid in focusing thought and becoming still. Practicing these still positions and/or exercises will put the mind even and Qi (energy) at rest; further, this practice can adjust the flow of blood and energy throughout the body and promote an attitude of purposeful discipline.

The purpose of "regulating the body," besides regulating the mind and breath by focusing the mind and calming the spirit, is most importantly to stabilize the circulation of blood and energy, to stretch the muscles, and to strengthen the bones. It is thus possible to rid the body of disease and extend life.

A basic imperative when trying to regulate the body is that the postures be correct and the body relaxed. Not only must the posture be correct, it must be maintained under all circumstances, whether walking, standing, sitting, lying, or doing work. If one's posture is not correct, the energy flow in the body will be obstructed and thought will be disrupted; and once the thought is unstill and the energy dispersed, health will be adversely affected.

Correct postures promote life. When still, one will have the dignified manner of one who knows one's place in the universe; when in movement, one will be agile, quick, and have great strength. A relaxed body is relaxed in the midst of tension, balancing strength and weakness, concerned with movement and stillness at the same time. One must be relaxed but not flaccid, taut but not stiff. The postures should be relaxed, but the thought should be concentrated; one should use thought, not power. If the posture is correct and the body relaxed, energy can flow naturally, and this is the best for health.

The human body can assume endless postures, which fall into four categories: walking, standing, sitting, and lying. In ancient times these were known as the "four majesties": "One should walk like the wind, stand like the pine, sit like a bell, lie like a bow." Proper postures and movement have always been an aid to good health; they allow the body to develop evenly, movement to be coordinated, the bodily form to be dignified and pleasing to the eyes, and in accordance with biological principles. They will increase the strength and effectiveness of the muscles and bones. A person with proper posture and movement will tire less easily and not easily be injured.

The art of walking includes practicing proper posture during everyday walks, the Hsing Bu (Step-by-Step) posture, and other postures. Those who practice Qigong walk notice the general condition of their surroundings and maintain their tranquility; they also focus upon the Dantian (a point about three inches below the navel, or in the lower abdomen), or the Ming Hsueh (an energy point). They relax the lower back and straighten up the spinal column; they stand upright and do not sway. Thus they are able to walk swiftly as the wind. Straightening out the arms and sticking out the chest are unnecessary; the whole body should be relaxed. The feet should be parallel, the heel of the foot should stride the ground first, and the ball of the foot should grasp the ground with force. This will increase the benefits of walking by increasing blood circulation throughout the body, and it will increase body strength in general.

At the same time one can regulate one's breath. While inhaling, pull up the stomach and tuck in the belly; when exhaling, relax the abdomen and waist, and try to focus energy on the Dantian. When walking, let the mind guide the energy, sending it to the center of the foot. This will increase blood circulation to the feet as well as to the head. Move lithely, lightly, and with agility. Moving in such a way is called "stepping like a monkey." The stomach will tighten up, strengthening the lower back and legs. This is especially beneficial for elderly people and those with high blood pressure.

The art of standing, also called standing firmly, evolved from ancient health traditions, Kung Fu, Nei Jia Quan (sect of internal practice of martial art), and other arts. The most basic standing form is the natural stance (figure 4). The feet should be parallel and the shoulders squared, the knees should be slightly bent but not extended past the tips of the toes. Pull up

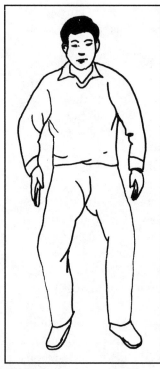

Fig. 4. Natural stance mode.

the groin muscles and tuck in the buttocks, straighten the lower back and relax the abdomen, hold the chest in close, stretch the back, relax the shoulders and the area under the arms. Let the shoulders droop a bit, let the wrists hang loose; let the arms hang naturally, and relax the front of the neck. Face the palm down with the fingers facing forward, curving and slightly separated naturally. Empty the mind while remaining alert. Look straight ahead and relax the eyelids, drooping them slightly. Focus the eyes inward or else fix them on a point far away. Close the mouth and slightly pull the teeth together, placing the tongue against the palate. And, of course, adjust the thought process and coordinate the breathing.

Raise the hands until the fingers point straight ahead, then deliberately press down with the palms. This is called the "pressing" form (figure 5). Raise the hands and make a motion as if pressing a ball that is floating on the water. Raise the arms no higher than breast level or lower than the navel. Curve the elbows as if about to hug something. This is called the "pressing the ball" form. Face the palms toward each other and raise the arms as if about to hug a tree trunk. This form is called "holding the ball" (figure 6).

Turn the feet slightly inward and position the fingers as if holding a ball (like a tiger's claws). This is the "triple curve" form, for the feet are curved,

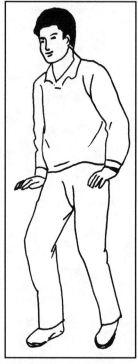

Fig. 5. The pressing form.

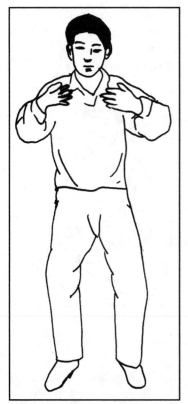

Fig. 6. Embracing ball (holding the ball) mode.

the arms are curved, and the hands are curved (figure 7). Depending on how strenuously you wish to exercise, you can adjust the height of your arms and the bending of your knees. It is important to keep in mind that the head should be held upright, with the neck straight; the nose should be at a point in a direct line above the navel; energy should be sent upward; and the bottoms of the feet should be firmly planted, with the legs as stable as trees rooted in the ground. Exhale like a goose alighting, and inhale like a bird taking flight—slowly and naturally, as though you were a flying spirit.

Standing exercise is best suited to those in relatively good health; it is useful as a fitness exercise and can cure many chronic diseases. It is especially helpful in treating high blood pressure, astigmatism, mental weakness, or nervousness.

Let us move onto sitting exercises. In ancient times much use was made of "stumble sitting" (also called "lotus sitting"), which is sitting with the legs crossed. One should be totally relaxed in order to be comfortable. When naturally crossing one's legs, the lower legs should be crossed forming an X with the feet underneath the thighs. The upper body

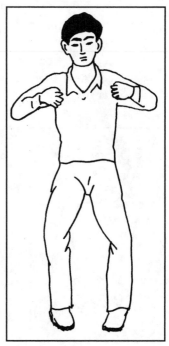

Fig. 7. Circle standing mode (triple-curve form).

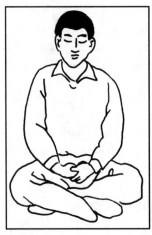

Fig. 8. Naturally cross-legged mode.

should be in the same position as if standing. In one position, called "palms together," the palms of the hands are clasped together, and the arms are held out in front of the chest (as if praying).

The "leaving an impression" (Tie Yin) position calls for the palms of the hands to be held upward, with the arms outstretched and the left on top of the right, and the thumbs opposite each other. In Buddhism these are called "intertwining hand postures" (Jie Shou Yin) (figure 8).

The single entwined knee position is achieved when one calf is placed on top of the other (figure 9). For the double entwined

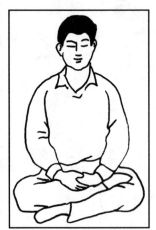

Fig. 9. Single cross-legged mode.

knee position, the left foot is first placed on top of the right leg and then the right is placed on the left leg, with the soles of both feet facing upward (figure 10).

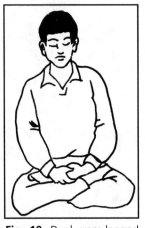

Fig. 10. Dual cross-legged mode.

These cross-legged positions, once achieved and held, are useful in helping people to achieve a peaceful, still frame of mind without leading to drowsiness. This is especially useful for people with circulatory problems whose heart muscles have been damaged. However, after a while most people find it uncomfortable to remain in these postures. When this is the case, one can utilize seated postures (see figure 11). Select a chair, stool, or bed of a comfortable height. Be seated with the feet flat on the floor and knees bent at a

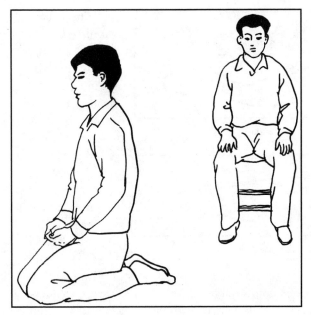

Fig. 11. Flat sitting mode.

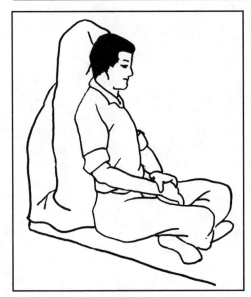

Fig. 12. Leaning sitting mode.

90-degree angle. The feet should be separated as far apart as the shoulders, the arms can hang naturally with the palms down on top of the thighs, or, as in the "leaving an impression" posture, with the palms on top of each other. Leaning sitting postures (figure 12) are useful for those who are weak or who have trouble with breathing or digestion.

We now turn to lying postures. The side posture in ancient times was known as the "Xiyi's sleeping" position (figure 13). Lying on the back was known as the "encircle the sun" position (figure 14).

If one prefers to lie on one's side, lying on the right side is better for the heart muscles; it also aids the liver in cleaning the blood and digesting the contents of the stomach. However, those afflicted with prolapse of gastric mucosa should avoid sleeping on the right side, in order to prevent the intestinal blockage caused by the prolapsed mucosa.

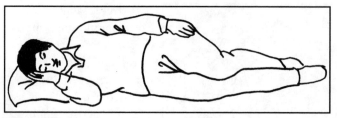

Fig. 13. Side sleeping mode (Xi Yi's sleeping position).

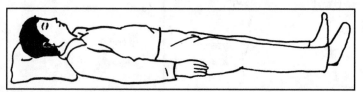

Fig. 14. Face-up sleeping mode (encircle the sun).

The pillow should be as high as the width of the shoulders. The head can extend a bit further from the end of the pillow, so that the neck can be relaxed. The hand of the raised part of the body should be placed comfortably on the hip, and the arm underneath the body should be naturally bent with the palm facing upward on the pillow. The back and groin area should be relaxed, and the trunk of the body should form a bow shape. The thigh under the body should be bent forward slightly, with the lower leg extending straight down. The leg on top should be bent making an angle of about 120 degrees, with the thigh and calf placed a little behind the lower leg underneath. One has the option of placing the palm of the upper hand in front of the lower abdomen. This helps to focus on the Dantian (the area below the navel and a source of Qi energy).

When lying on one's back, one can either lie flat or use a pillow to raise the back to form an angle called the "vigorous style." The arms and legs should be extended naturally, but should be straight and relaxed. The palms should face down and be placed alongside the trunk, or the fingers should be curved into an empty fist. The feet can be spaced comfortably apart or the ankles can be crossed.

Lying exercises are useful for weak patients or for practicing before sleep. Half-reclining exercises are good for those with heart trouble or breathing difficulties.

Qigong exercises performed while lying on the side or back will enable those with physical deformities or injuries to achieve mobility. However, it is easy to fall asleep while practicing Qigong in lying positions. They are not beneficial to those in good health, or who want to increase their physical strength.

In conclusion, in practicing Qigong, to each his own. There are methods and levels suitable for all times and places and physical states that will invigorate the body and maintain the health of all organs and systems.

When participating in any kind of physical activity, it is important to change body positions frequently and adjust the strenuousness of the exercise (the balance between tension and relaxation) to a reasonable and comfortable level to avoid overexertion.

Regulate breathing to cultivate Qi

To regulate breathing is to strengthen energy by adjusting and controlling one's inhaling and exhaling. This is done to achieve the cultivation of genuine Qi, a pure heart, and a calm spirit. The main idea can be expressed as: (1) blow out, (2) yawn, and (3) spit out; (4) draw in, (5) to raise, (6) to lower, (7) to open, (8) to close.

This is different from simply breathing deeply or following other breathing exercises, as it is combined with the idea of regulating the mind. This intertwined idea makes the examination of the method and results most compelling.

In ancient times disciplined breathing exercises were known as "Tuna" (exhaling and inhaling). The basic methods were not particularly difficult to learn, but the inappropriate use will result in the deviation of effect, especially in the practice of the ancient ways of "sending Qi," "dispersing Qi," "transferring Qi," and "methods of heaven cycles." One must be very careful when beginning a study of breathing exercises. One must have a good teacher to put one on the right track during the initial learning period. This cannot be learned from books or by oneself.

The purpose of regulating breath is to focus thought in order to become still. One can use breathing to balance "Yin" and "Yang" (two opposite aspects in the body), to coordinate the functioning of body systems, to stimulate existing physical attributes, and to improve total physical condition.

Modern scientific investigation has concluded that breath regulation strengthens the functions of heart, lung, stomach, and intestines; improves organs' blood circulation; is useful in adjusting the metabolism; and increases the body's storage of energy.

Breath regulation is done as follows: Using normal breath as the basis of breath regulation, gradually use this progression: uniform, precise, calm, long. Naturally there are other requirements, such as that one should breathe like the wind, enunciating a word while breathing (like "om"). The former is the most common requirement to achieve a state of calmness. There is an old saying, "The heart is calm, the breath even." "Cultivate the breath that gives life"; this is useful for health and longevity, the opposite being "(His) energy is scattered and the heart is disturbed," which is very bad for health.

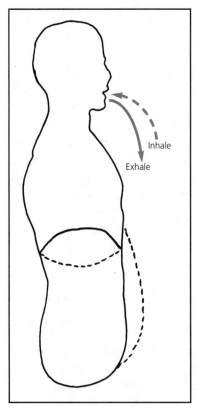

The latter method may be used to rid the body of bad energy and to build up good energy, which is beneficial to the special disorders of the inner organs.

"Regulating breath" is only two words, but takes many forms.

1. Use of mouth and nose. Usually one breathes through the nose. But if the chest is stuffy and full and breathing is difficult, one may use the nose to breathe in and the mouth to breathe out. As to help cure diseases of the inner organs, such as the exercise known as "Six-Word Formula," which emphasizes deep breathing, one may also use the mouth to breathe out and nose to breathe in. If one has a cold or if the nose is obstructed by other diseases, one may use the mouth to breathe in and out.

2. Use of various muscles in breathing. As a general rule, abdominal breathing is the best. This goes along with biological requirements and is the basic method of regulating breath to increase energy.

Fig. 15. Belly (abdominal) breathing.

As infants, most people will use the abdominal muscles to breathe or combine abdominal and chest muscles to breathe. When one is inhaling, the diaphragm is pulled downward; pressure increases in the abdomen and the abdomen expands. When one breathes out, the diaphragm rises naturally, and the abdominal muscles contract. Male adults mainly use abdominal breathing (figure 15); women mainly use chest breathing (figure 16). Those trained in a particular art, such as athletes, martial artists, or singers, use abdominal breathing.

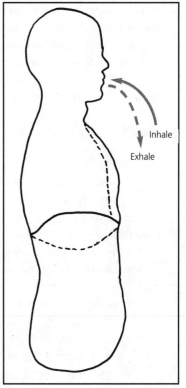

Fig. 16. Chest breathing.

Chest breathing mainly uses rib muscles, with the chest moving as one breathes in and out. This type of breathing is comparatively shallow unless one is consciously trying to take deep breaths. After a heavy meal or if something is pressing on the abdomen, or if the abdomen is distended, one can use chest breathing and be a bit more comfortable. Abdominal/chest breathing is a combination of both, in which both areas follow breathing, so this is called "complete inhalation." When breathing deeply, to expand the capacity of the lungs, one should use this method. Abdominal breathing is known as "natural breathing." Chest breathing is called "reverse breathing."

If one intends to use abdominal muscles to aid in breathing exercises, then while exhaling one uses force in contracting the abdominal muscles; this is called "assisted abdominal breathing."

When one is inhaling and contracts the abdominal area, and when exhaling one relaxes the abdominal muscles, this is called "opposing abdominal breathing."

These two types of abdominal breathing both have effects on the chest and abdominal cavities and, because of this, may have the effect of gently massaging various internal organs and improving circulation to these organs. Assisted abdominal breathing is useful in cultivating Qi and the opposite abdominal breathing is more used in "heaven cycle" exercises.

Controlling breathing with the mind

Usually most people take no notice of their breathing, which is taken for granted and is known as "natural breathing." This really does not qualify to be called regulated breathing, and yet it really is breathing that is regulated by itself, as this is the type of breathing unconsciously done by the body when it is most relaxed. When one is calm and at peace, the breathing you do is called "still breathing." Breathing is a process which is inextricably related to a person's activity level and emotions.

When one is beginning the study of Qigong and one becomes too anxious about one's breathing and tries to consciously alter it, the rhythm misses the point entirely—breathing will become a burden on one's mind and produce unnecessary nervousness to the degree that breathing will become irregular. The secret is to focus one's concentration on normal breathing, follow its natural rhythm, only paying attention to one's inhaling and exhaling, as if thought and breath were one. This is known as "following one's breath method"; just paying attention to one's breathing, not trying to alter it.

If one tries to count one's breaths from one to ten or one to one hundred, paying attention to the whole cycle, practice exhaling and count exhalations, practice inhaling and count inhalations, this is called "counting breath method." One can concentrate one's thoughts on one's breathing and not allow one's mind to be distracted. A novice may also calmly listen to the sound of one's own breathing to improve concentration. This is known as the "listen to breath method." After one becomes thoroughly familiar with these methods, one may reach a point when one's breathing becomes very deep, slow, and soft, where it is controlled but not directed, where breathing is almost imperceptible. This is known as "breath stopping."

When one is well advanced in breath regulation, it is possible to direct Qi (bodily energy), to move it around. This is the step of "using thought to direct Qi." "Where one's thought goes, so does Qi." This is called "moving Qi," as in "move the Qi to Dantian," which is during deep abdominal breathing, to direct the "Qi" to the lower abdomen below the navel. If one is practicing opposed abdominal breathing, when one is exhaling, the lower abdomen may be pushed out and downward. This is called "Qi sinking into Dantian."

The next step is to imagine breath is coming in and out through the navel. This is known as "navel breathing," or "Dantian breathing," or "congenital breathing." If it really appears as if breathing is really being done through the navel and not through the nose or mouth, and is therefore as delicate as to be almost not noticed, this is known as "fetal breathing." The test of this "fetal breathing" is, if a feather is held up to the nose and the feather does not move. This is a sort of very deep abdominal breathing, described by Laotze as "it is as if one can continue forever, using this but not exhausting it."

This is an extension of closing the breath. Appearing as if one's breath has stopped, one can find oneself imagining that breath is coming in and out through the navel. If we go one step further and have a suggestion that breathing had stopped, one may imagine that breath is coming in and out through the pores of the body; like the movements of clouds or fog. This is called "pore breathing," "body breathing," or "open and closed breathing." Open and closed breathing is described as when inhaling, air is absorbed through the Dantian from outside the body, then the pores are closed; when exhaling it seems as if air is being expelled through the Dantian. The pores simultaneously open everywhere on the body except the head area.

To take this to still another level, in "real Qi" as breath rises and falls, the Qi travels through the meridians of the entire body; or else rises when inhaling and falls when exhaling; or falls during inhalation and rises during exhalation; or rises during one inhalation and exhalation; or falls during one inhalation and exhalation. Perhaps during one inhalation and exhalation, it travels through one meridian or only a part, so to finish one meridian every few breaths. The Qi may travel in a circular movement, or it may travel in a straight line. It may stop for a time at the original place and hover there. This is all called "moving the Qi (energy)." The so-called heel breath method which is moving Qi to the heel of the foot when

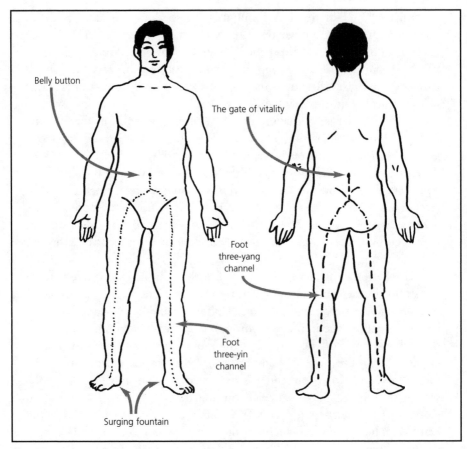

Belly button

The gate of vitality

Foot
three-yang
channel

Foot
three-yin
channel

Surging fountain

Fig. 17. Heel exercise method.

beginning a breath, as you breathe in you move the energy up in the Yang meridians on the posterior and internal aspects of the legs (a "meridian" is a term used in traditional Chinese medicine to describe an energy pathway through the body) to meet at the Mingmen (vital gate) point (around the second lumbar vertebra at the back) and then to middle Dantian (umbilicus). When exhaling, one moves the Qi in Ren meridian (on the midline of the chest/abdomen) down to the Huiyin (perineum), then splits the energy into two parts going down each inner leg following the Yin meridians to the sole of the foot at Yongquan point (rising spring) (figure 17).

Or, in some cases this is done without thinking the inhalation or exhalation: one may send the energy from Dantian to Yongquan or the heel of the foot. In the book *Qigong Liao Fa Shi Jian* (*Qigong Therapy in Practice*) is described the "nine-breath method," a form of directing breathing. You must imagine your body to be completely transparent and the spinal column as having three circulatory pathways, beginning at Yintang point (an energy point between the eyebrows) and ending at Huiyin (perineum). The center pathway was thought to be as thick as a reed, the outside blue, the inside red. The pathways to the right and left were as thick as a wheat stalk, the left was white and the right red. For the exercise one first used the left ring finger (in Chinese, the no-name finger) to block the left nostril; one then inhaled through the right nostril and let the air/energy travel from Yintang back down the right circulatory pathway to behind Huiyin; from there it should pass to the left pathway and travel up to Yintang and out through the nose. This should be repeated three times, and then use the left nostril in the same manner to circulate through the left pathway first back up through the right three times and then use both nostrils to breathe in, down the side two circulatory pathways up behind Huiyin, unite and enter the central pathway up and out the nose, three times. For this reason it is called "nine-breath method." (See figure 18.) After one has practiced this method thoroughly it is not necessary to

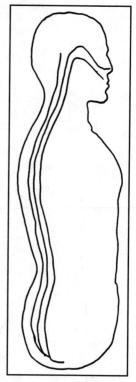

Fig. 18. Nine-breath method.

block the nostrils: one can direct pure life-giving energy from the air of the environment into one's body to flush out poisons and disease-bearing elements and so make the body pure and shining, "the central spinal circulatory path (Du meridian) red as rouge and bright as a lamp, soft as a lotus petal and as straight as a palm tree trunk." This method is a Tantric

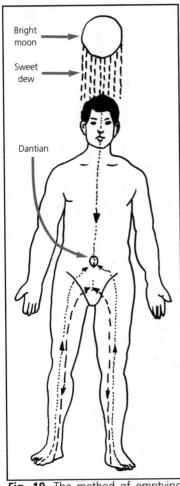

Bright
moon

Sweet
dew

Dantian

Fig. 19. The method of emptying into Dantian (the public region).

Buddhist tradition known as "nine points wind," a preparatory exercise for the "illumination of the mind where the spirit can leave the body (open the top door)." Actually this is the combination of imagination and breath.

The so-called Dantian halt energy method was a mind exercise in which you imagine there is a bright shining full moon above your head which slowly dissipates into a colorful fog which seeps into Du meridian at the top and travels down to Huiyin, splits in two and travels down the leg to the sole of the foot, expelling all pain and worry as it goes. The body and mind are relaxed and happy; then one imagines the fog travels upward from the sole to Dantian and stops to merge with descending fog from the top as if one had two vases inverted on each other, capturing the air not exhaling, the longer the better until you cannot bear it any longer, then slowly exhale through the nose but leaving some energy air in the Dantian area, then direct some of this air through Du meridian (the central energy pathway) up through the top of the pathway and out. (See figure 19.) This type of exercise with breath-holding was called "Chan style method" (Chan was a school of meditative Buddhism) in the Tang dynasty book *Prescriptions Worth 1,000 Pieces of Gold*, and was thought to bring about a glowing complexion; soft, healthy hair; alert hearing and keen sight; a good appetite and strength; and a cure for all ailments in general. This method could have been derived from the Tantric *Precious Vessel Qi*, they are quite similar. A practice known as "Xiao zhou tian" (minor heaven cycle), or "Huo Che Ban Yun" is moving pure Qi (energy) and upward through the "Du" meridian and pass alongside the "Ren" meridian downward (front midline). (See figures 20–22.)

One cycle is thought to be one trip around the heavens. The "major heaven cycle" method is causing Qi energy to pass through many channels (meridians) in the body (the eight extra-ordinary and twelve regular meridians) at intervals coordinated to breathing. (See figure 23.)

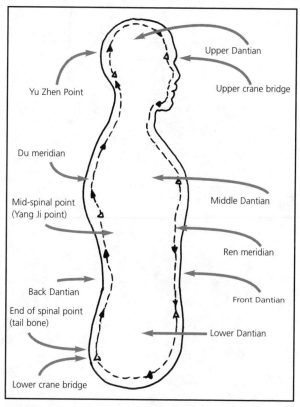

Upper Dantian

Yu Zhen Point

Upper crane bridge

Du meridian

Mid-spinal point (Yang Ji point)

Middle Dantian

Ren meridian

Back Dantian

Front Dantian

End of spinal point (tail bone)

Lower Dantian

Lower crane bridge

Fig. 20. Minor circuit Gong (minor heaven cycle).

Coordinating movement in Qigong practice

The most common admonition for the body position in Qigong exercises is tongue position. Most often one is told to hold the tongue against the roof of the mouth, or else force-fully roll back the tongue against the soft palate. This increases production of saliva. In one exercise, one moves one's tongue in this way thirty-six times to produce saliva and then swallows it in three gulps, coordinating breathing to send it to the Dantian. Most times when breathing in the tongue should be held against the roof of the mouth and relaxed while exhaling. This is useful to fix concentration and achieve calm

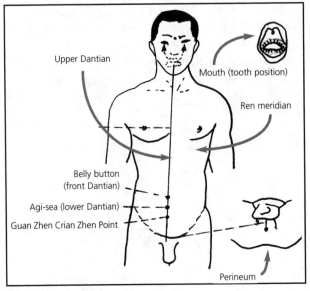

Fig. 21. Minor circuit Gong (minor heaven cycle).

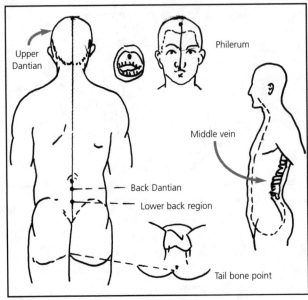

Fig. 22. Minor circuit (minor heaven cycle).

(or stasis). While practicing the "Zhou tian" exercises, one should tighten the anus and pull in the stomach. When exhaling relax the stomach and muscles of the anal/crotch area.

Even when not practicing "Zhou tian" exercise, it is a good idea to contract one's anus muscles when doing any kind of breathing exercise. This will be useful in remedying internal organ prolapse, or hemorrhoids caused by insufficiency of Qi.

In "assisted abdominal breathing," one relaxes one's abdomen and perineum when breathing in and tighten them when breathing out.

A simple coordination of movement may be known as "rising falling," "opening closing." In general, breathing in is associated with rising and falling movement, such as standing up tall and drawing inward. Exhaling and downward movements are coordinated with postures of relaxation and openness (see figures 24–26). For therapeutic use: For those suffering from symptoms indicating excessive "Yang" in the body (an example is high blood pressure) one should make use of postures of falling and openness. For maladies of weakness or cold in the body, postures of rising and closure are best (an

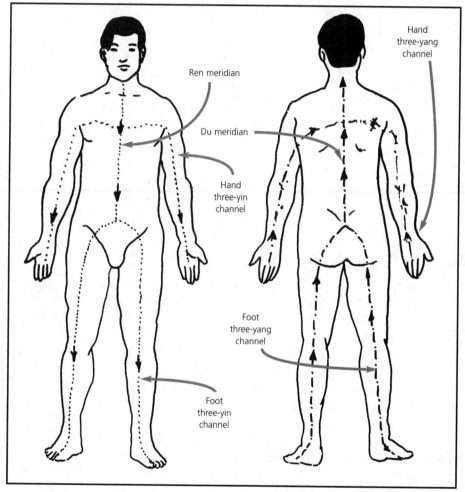

Fig. 23. Major circuit Gong (major heaven cycle).

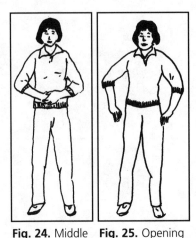

Fig. 24. Middle   **Fig. 25.** Opening
Dantian   mode.
breathing.

**Up-down opening-closing
breathing method**

example of weakness would be low blood pressure). These guidelines are not absolute. When trying to coordinate regulation of the body, mind, and will, you may have to employ falling in the midst of rising, and openness with closure, so each is measured and governed by its opposite. One must be flexible and use whatever degree works best for the individual case.

Whole systems of coordinated breathing and movement have become quite numerous, such as the "new Qigong," "breathing from middle Dantian," "opening and closing Dantian," natural breathing or "wind," breathing in slow and accelerated styles, Ma Litang six–character rule style, Qin Chongsan five–element palm exercise, and the ancient eight-section Jin tradition, to mention a few.

Reciting a mantra

This may take the form of uttering words or simply making a sound. The most often seen is "inner cultivation method" mantras. One may choose a word or phrase which best exemplifies one's goal in one's progress to better health, the length of the utterance depends on the deepness of the breathing. Initially, a student may select "peaceful," "relaxation," "happiness," or as one's breath is shallow and split the phrase into two parts, breathing in and then out. Later, as one becomes more advanced, more words are added. These words themselves can become a sort of "timer" for the length of a breath. In this way these mantras can have a calming effect on breathing, help the regulation of breath and serve as psychological cues to have a positive benefit to one's physiology. In ancient times the "six word rule" put a great

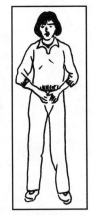

Fig. 26.
Closing mode.

emphasis on breathing out. One was able to rid one's body of malevolent Qi and regulate the function of the liver, heart, spleen, kidneys, and lungs. Diseases caused by excess heat in the body were cured by mantras, selecting one of six words—"hsu," "ho," "hu," "si," "chui" (or "whistle"), "hsi"—pronounced while breathing out, the emphasis being in the form of the mouth rather than the sound. One can also select one sound according to the season—in spring "hsu," summer "ho," autumn "si," in winter "chui" ("whistle"); or one may use each formation in succession— but take care not to overdo the exercise either in duration or intensity.

The use of mantras became known as "Tu Yin (literally, pronouncing sound) Dao Yin," classed under "eliminating" methods, useful in diseases where accumulations of unwanted heat, Qi, or other bodily products needed to be gotten rid of. One can move Qi around to various parts of the body, for example, clean the liver to help all other functions of digestion and beauty. Wu Shu (Kung fu) artists use these methods to increase strength, singers can use these methods in vocal exercises, poets can use these exercises to promote clarity and resonance in their speech—all are a sort of "Tu Yin Dao Yin" (movement of Qi by means of sound-pronunciation) discipline.

Proper length of breath—specifically, how does one decide the proper length of time for one breath?

If one is trying to adjust the Yin and Yang, heat and cold in the body (for a good balance of natural metabolic functions), one can do breath control. In general, one should concentrate on breathing in, extending the time taken breathing in, depth of inhalation and pause, and hold the breath when one wishes to build up the Yang functions and get rid of "cold" in the body. (Cold problems typically have to do with rheumatism, diarrhea, etc.) Conversely, if one wishes to build up the Yin and eliminate excess of heat, one concentrates on exhalation, lengthening its duration, taking care to expel all air, and pausing before taking the next breath. (Problems with excess of heat can be seen through skin irritations, headache, etc.)

"Pause breathing" is of three types. The first is breathe-in breath-out—pause. This is also called "soft breathing method." The sequence breathe in–pause–breathe out is called "hard breathing method."

The sequence inhale-pause-inhale-exhale is rarely practiced and is considered a type of inhalation exercise. The pauses in breathing should not be so long that one has the feeling of obstructing one's breathing. Ancient books mention "extremes of breath-stoppage," which really was holding one's breath until one could not endure this state any longer. Indeed, sick people should be very wary of attempting any regimen of breath control without a physician's advice.

"Long and deep breathing" proceeds from normal breathing gradually becoming light, calm, even, and long with practice until the practitioner breathes three to four times a minute or even one to two times a minute or until breathing is imperceptible and called "embryo breathing." "Shallow short breathing" or "larynx breathing" is an aberration of beginners, especially those with illness, and it should be corrected.

Zhuang Zi does mention in one of his books, "supreme people breathe with their throats," so special cases of people with certain diseases may use this type of breathing as normal breathing.

Speed of breathing

Taking normal breathing as a starting point, one gradually moderates one's breathing to make it slower, softer, and more even, the so-called calm breathing method. The other forms, "embryo breathing," "heel breathing," "open closed breathing," and others, all are forms of slow deep breathing. In special cases, abrupt, short, noisy breathing is used. This is the so-called wind breathing. Ancient books proscribe this method, saying "gathered wind will dissipate," but using this method to rid the body of abnormal conditions can have very positive results.

In "new Qigong therapy," "wind breathing" is used to alleviate many chronic diseases—even bringing some forms of cancer into remission. These patients' breathing is usually shallow—so at the start of practice, the quick shallow breathing (wind breathing) is actually more natural to them. Repeated short shallow inhaling or exhaling, known as "halting breath" or "Qi," is used extensively by those practicing "inner Kung fu." When concentrating one's strength at a certain point, one exhales suddenly, emitting a sound (commonly known as a ki-ai). Some people study in the "Yi Jin Jing" (changing muscles tract), which is associated with sudden, explosive exhalation for building strength.

Regulate the Mind and Adjust Thought

The basis for this can be summed up quite simply. "Concentration," or from another viewpoint, all ideas are focused on one point and keep one's focus on that point. All one's effort should be directed on one thing, and one may practice imagining things, too. In ancient times this was called "keeping the thought," "keeping the idea," "keeping the spirit," "viewing a point," "meditation," "reflection," "stop one's view," "focusing one's mind," etc. This exercise in thought is essentially being able to focus, rid one's mind of stray, unrelated thought, to avoid distraction.

Regulating thought also encompasses "living life in a calm and purposeful manner." This is the way to health and long life. If one keeps one's emotions under control, then Qi can flow evenly (and not become displaced or blocked). One will have sufficient energy and spirit which builds upon itself for a happy long life. That is to say, regulating the mind can have an effect on blood and Qi (energy) circulation which affects the function of body organs. Mind, therefore, leads Qi which flows through the body and invigorates the blood. In this state the Yin will be even and the Yang under control—the organs will work together harmoniously. Modern medical investigation indicates that psychological factors play a vital but indefinable role in good health. If one has a healthy mental attitude, then one will have good health in general "to bring about change," "to realize" which will have definite effect on one's physical and mental condition. One must focus one's energy and take an objective look at oneself, then with an even, optimistic attitude do all in one's power to gradually and realistically discipline one's mind and habits and bring them into line with a healthful way of living. One can see that regulating the mind is a central tenet of Qigong and really a crucial aspect for healthy living in general.

The significance of regulating the mind is to protect the body as "the house of royalty"; to avoid disturbance by outside matters or things, to keep the spirit free and clear and the Qi fresh. When one's thoughts are clear, one is at peace.

Real experience has proved that thought can control some processes of the involuntary nervous system. If one can control one's thoughts and become calm, one can adjust many physiological capabilities.

The purpose of regulating the mind can be stated in two words: "become calm." Thoughts should be channeled into a calm attitude. "Calmness" or "statis" was originally a Taoist term, indicating going to a quiet place, clear one's mind and meditate, without personal thought or direction. Buddhism calls this state "chan ding" (deep meditation), Confucianism "zuo wang" (sitting and forgetting), "gathering of the mind"—these are all alike, and the object is to arrive at a state of calm contemplation, forgetting one's self. The Chinese medical book *Simple Questions—Ancient True Theory*, describes a state "peaceful," "clear," and "empty," "clear" meaning innocent and simple, and "empty" meaning not motivated by ambition or desire. This emptiness serves to teach the will—the innocence teaches the spirit.

As any Kung Fu has various states and levels so does calmness have various degrees—at very least we can divide it into three levels. When one begins to practice Qigong, one should not be too strict about becoming calm; worrying about it would make it impossible to calm down. At the beginning just approach the matter with a clear heart and gradually rid one's mind of stray thoughts. If one can just focus one's concentration for a time, this is enough. An ancient saying, "Do not be worried about thoughts arising; only be concerned about keeping awareness sharp." Realizing that stray thoughts are popping up is the first step in clearing them out. At this stage calmness will be a struggle between clearheadedness and miscellaneous thoughts; regulating one's mind will be a conscious effort, but one which must be done gently.

When one becomes more practiced in meditation, thoughts intrude less often, the mind more regulated. This stage of "concentration of mind" is partly conscious, partly unconscious, completely natural. At this stage one is prone to all sorts of feelings and imaginings, such as "Ba Chu" (enter into an emotional state—like rapture), "sixteen environments," etc.

The final state is reached when one achieves "Nothingness." At this stage the mind is still as a mirror—water clear and calm—without thoughts or worries yet knowing all with no separation between self and outside but able to distinguish between the two. The spirit completely alert—one reaches an "empty soul" state. "Quiet without movement, feelings pass through."

Methods and experiences in regulating the mind are rich and the only method is "concentration of mind," but types and style vary. To combat intruding thoughts one must recognize them as they arise and have reasonable training in dealing with them. This is not simply an effort to supress thought but as in "An Introduction to Medicine—Health Preservation" is said "When you understand the reason, you will have no more longings and your heart is clear and spirit happy; not to strive after calmness, but achieving it naturally." One can see that being patient and tolerant in one's moral philosophy, controlling one's wants and emotions, cultivating one's thought processes are the basis for regulating one's mind.

In order to prepare oneself to enter a state of calmness, one must, at least, do the following three exercises:

1. Try to set aside all types of troubling matters so one is not worried about anything. If one is very distracted by worries, one should not force oneself to practice meditation but try some soothing music or some aid like counting beads or the like to distance oneself.

2. Loosen one's clothing and go to the bathroom if needed, to make oneself comfortable as possible.

3. Select the most peaceful surroundings you can find—and fix oneself at an appropriate place. Some may wish to put up a sign or light a stick of incense. Try to make your surroundings, time, and conditions for meditation regular. All aspects will have an influence and you are more likely to succeed in your efforts.

"Concentation of mind" methods vary but are the same in three aspects.

1. One focuses one's concentration on one part of the body and observes all feelings or states of that place.
2. Notice some functions of the body and try to regulate it.
3. Imagine some good thing or action which would serve as a cue.

"Focusing inward" means concentrating on either "Qi" points, meridians, certain limbs, or internal organs. The most common "centering" point is the "lower Dantian" (see figures 20–22). In general this is thought to be slightly below the navel. Concentrating on this point can send Qi to its base or "home," if one wishes to send Qi to other places or organs, it is the place to start. "Upper Dantian" is behind the Qi point Yintang (which is between the eyebrows), below the Baihui point (at the center of the top of the head), in the center of the brain. Focusing thought on this point is good for increasing knowledge and improving brain function. But this should be avoided by those with Qi accumulated in the upper body. "Middle Dantian" is at the Danzhong point or behind the navel in front of the lower back, but the location varies in interpretation. This is useful for centering Qi to improve digestion or appetite.

"Anterior Dantian" is in the navel. Centering here can improve digestive organs and aid in body development. "Posterior Dantian" is at the second lumbar vertebra (the Mingmen point), can improve the kidneys (which is considered as the congenital foundation of the body in TCM), and strengthen the Yang. Other Qi points such as Qihai, Huiyin, Yongquan are often used to focus and strengthen Qi and nourish the Yin. Focusing on meridians (energy pathways) is the way of active suggestion of mind concentration, often used in the heavens cycle exercises, which is focusing on the circulation of Ren and Du meridians. Also used are the Dai and Yinqiao and Yangqiao meridians. Any of the eight extra and twelve regular meridians can be used for centering of mind. "Heel breathing," "nine breaths method," described earlier, etc., are all focusing thought methods using meridians. Centering the mind on a disease is possible and is mentioned in ancient tracts (as in focusing on the source of the disease), but should only be undertaken under a doctor's care. There is the danger of increasing the severity of the disease. The point is to move Qi toward or away from that point to speed the recovery.

Focusing on a limb of the body is used in relaxation exercises, standing meditation, or active exercises. Focusing on one's breath is the most commonly used method, like the counting of breaths, sending Qi to Dantian exercises described earlier. Focusing on inner organs is also known as "reflecting the light of the spirit," "looking inward," etc. The so-called receiving interior scenes is a kind of imaginary centering. As in "plain question" records. First imagine the heart as a red sun, Qi as crimson energy flowing from it, going "south upward" becoming a bright ball of fire; green Qi emanates from the liver, traveling on the east (left), becoming a bright green forest. Not only do the five inner organs give out five colors of Qi, but a great "North Star" is over the head. "When Proper Qi is held within, evil cannot disturb it." In the Siu dynasty book *Theory of the Origin of All Disease* is also mentioned "Qi of the heart is crimson; of the liver, green; of the lungs, white; of the spleen, yellow; and of the kidneys, black. This shines throughout the body."

The Tang dynasty tract *Detailed Precious Prescriptions (1,000 Gold)*, mentions that one should often practice the "Yellow Emperor's inner reflection method" in order to cultivate one's health. This was like looking into one's inner organs which were like variegated stone—five colors can be distinguished. The "Precious Prescription," "Chan Reflective Method," was a kind of exercise borrowed from forms of Qigong mental control methods. One was to imagine that Tai He Yuan (original) Qi was descending in the form of a purple cloud—like a cover—five colors then becoming visible which seep into the body through the skin from head to toe, flowing through the limbs and inner organs. If one practices this three to five times a day, all diseases will be eliminated.

One can perform mental regulation exercises while doing physical or still Qigong exercise, perhaps accompanied by appropriate postures. One can imagine one is floating on water, holding a ball, carrying water, stirring mud, fighting a tiger, pushing a mountain, supporting the heavens, doing martial arts, or dancing. Without exerting much physical energy, but using mental energy, it is possible to circulate Qi and invigorate the blood, exercise the bones and muscles, and increase one's strength.

"Keeping the Outside," also called concentrating on the outside environment, means first noting the external environment and then closing one's eyes and imagining this picture; or one may imagine a particularly inviting scene of one's choosing. One may concentrate on still objects or still forms on a painting, or one may imagine moving scenes as in a movie. There is a kind of "Concentrate One's Thoughts on a Scene Method" whereby one looks intently on a particular scene and then one closes one's eyes and remembers it—this clears out stray extraneous thoughts, improves one's sight and memory. "Collect Beauty of the Day" and "Inhale the Magnificence of the Moon" methods are of this type.

The Taoist book *Cloud Curtain Seven Notes* speaks of face the sun when it is rising or setting, take nine gulps of air and hold them. Raise one's head, breathe in the sun's light, and swallow it nine times. This is good for the Yang (positive) function of the body. This is also called "Hsia Mu Sing Qi Fa" (Sunset Curtain Circulate Qi Method). When the moon appears, rises, and sets, face the moon, gulp air, and hold it eight times, raise your head, breathe in the gleaming moonbeams, and swallow them eight times. This stimulates the Yin (negative) function of the body. This is also called "Weng Yue Ching

Fa" (Bark at the Moon Method). Whether it is a memory or the imagination that lifts one's spirits or puts one in a dreamlike state, it all serves the purpose to enable one to achieve calmness and is beneficial to health.

Most people think focusing on the external is not as useful as focusing on the internal; but in the early stages of Qigong study, it is easier to focus on the external and to rid oneself of the many stray thoughts which intrude at this time. It is a useful first step. Repeating a phrase, something related to good health, the goal one is striving toward, is also a powerful stimulant. In Pavlovian theory, this is a "secondary system" stimulant. This is a personal suggestive type of focus and the content can be extremely varied; internal, external, moving, still, all can be chosen according to the disease, such as repeating "Relax," "Happiness," "Warmth," "Cold," "Heavy," "Power," "Lightness," "Countenance Bright and Glowing," "Beauty of Spring."

Verbal instruction by another person is a more concrete stimulation. Beginners and those who find it difficult to relax can achieve better results in much less time if a teacher guides them by word or if a tape is played, although the contents of the instruction should be chosen according to the person and/or their disease. This is guided and cued focusing. If direct stimulation of the senses is used to guide the practitioner to achieve calmness, this is considered guided focusing. Besides the cuing methods described above, using landscape or words, one can also use soft music, rhythm, poems, harmony, or chords. Whatever induces people to calm down, happily, in an artistic style, can be used to guide people. Buddhist monks use this when they keep time on "wooden fish," beat on drums or chimes, play religious music, intone scripture, or recite spells. Besides their religious significance, these guide people to a calm state, allowing them to leave aside other thoughts. Other devices such as incense, heat, cold, or massage, direct stimulation are all used to aid the novice achieve calmness.

If one compares movement and stillness, it is easier for novices to concentrate on movement, and it is better to concentrate on movement in the initial phases—one focuses on postures and movements when one studies still exercises; one can imagine moving exercises and use one's thought rather than one's strength, as in the "Yi Chin Ching," "Dragging Nine Oxen Tails," and really can cultivate Qi and increase strength—useful for weak persons or those unused to physical activity.

Focusing on the outside environment, things, or pictures such as running water, breezes, swings, a floating object, or other images, are classified as active focusing, can stimulate vitality, and make it easy to go into a reverie.

Focusing inward in small or greater circling the heaven exercise is also active focusing, can bring the Ying and Yang functions into balance, and promote circulation of blood and Qi throughout the body. But one must have a definite time to practice these exercises, or else one risks mistake or aberrations occurring.

Calm or meditative focusing, although somewhat more difficult to learn, is more suitable for those who are exhausted, or have weak Yin and excessive Yang. One may focus on inner or external meditative subjects. This can also relieve nervous conditions.

The goal of focusing is to eliminate the need for focusing. It is only a way of making people enter a calm state, so one should not concentrate on this exclusively. One should focus, then relax, gather one's energy and disperse it until one is focusing, but yet not until one can enter a meditative state without effort. After practicing for a time one will gradually achieve effortless regulation.

Using a Pavlovian explanation, one has established a conditional response when one arrives at a particular surrounding at a particular time; with familiar movements or positions one will naturally become calm. This is genuine skill. The level of the ability to achieve calmness is not so high as to be unattainable by ordinary people; one must only be regular, persistent. One will be successful. "Skill will come in time."

To illustrate the processes of therapy using the "Three Regulations" described above, we list below some common Qigong exercises:

1. Positions—natural crossed legs, single crossed legs, double crossed legs, standing (including strong standing), and free form—five types. The first four positions have been described earlier under "Regulating the Body" (figures 6–10). Free form does not impose any set position—one can practice any time, any place; one must only concentrate on relaxing the entire body, regulate one's breathing, and focus on the Dantian region.

2. Breathing. There is the calm breathing method, deep breathing, and reverse breathing. Calm breathing follows one's natural breathing and is suitable for beginners. Deep breathing and coordinating abdominal breathing have been described earlier. Reverse breathing and reverse ab-

dominal breathing have also been described; one must proceed with the last two with care, in the proper order; one should not force progress.

It is most important to focus on the small Dantian Area, 1.5 cm below the navel. Menstruating women should focus on the "middle" Dantian, which is located between the breast in the middle of the chest. Those with low blood pressure can also focus on the "Upper" Dantian, a point behind the mid-eyebrows, midbrain (see figure 20).

Strong Qigong practice is often indicated in the prevention or cure of neuroasthenia, cardioneurosis, dysfunction of autonomous nerve system, cerebroarteriosclerosis, hypertension, hypotension, coronary heart disease, myocardiac disorders, pulmonary tuberculosis, aplastic anemia, hyperthyroidism, dysfunctional uterine bleeding, chronic nephritis, renal tuberculosis, etc. Exercises and breathing and focusing methods are selected as indicated by the individual patient's condition. One usually should practice two or three times a day for thirty to sixty minutes.

In order to prevent unwanted results from one's Qigong practice, one must adhere to the following principles:

1. Process must be natural.
2. It must involve the entire body.
3. One must be self-motivated.
4. One must practice regularly.
5. Try to progress at a slow but steady rate.

One should at the same time embrace the following requirements:

1. Relaxation and tension, in turn should be natural.
2. One should practice both active and still exercises.
3. Emotions should be at peace, breath even.
4. The senses should be directed inward.
5. The mind and breath should be one.
6. Breath should be even and natural.
7. One should be relaxed but not flaccid; taut but not stiff.
8. One should hang the head slightly; pull in the chin; stretch the back while relaxing the chest, shoulders, and wrists; curve the elbows a bit to loosen the underarms; relax lower back but tighten the buttocks.

The knees should be slightly bent, feet evenly spaced. Internal condition should be coordinated with the external postures. The upper-lower body should coordinate. One should be attentive but not force oneself. One should be correct and peaceful.

Have a regular regimen of exercise and a set time to practice it.

Modern Scientific Investigation into Qigong Theory

Beginning in the 1950s, members of the Chinese medical profession have undertaken a wide-ranging experimental investigation and clinical observation of Qigong therapy. Within the limitations of the overview, I will attempt to describe some of their findings.

Modern investigation indicates that Qigong has definite effect of regulating the functions of the human body, and sometimes the adjustment is bi-directional. The practice of Qigong can strengthen the functions of nervous, endocrine, circulatory, digestive, respiratory, urinary, reproductive, and motoring systems, and improve metabolism to enable the body to remain in the status of low-consumption but high-reservation of energy, so is beneficial to the recovery from disease and extension of life span.

Concentration of mind and entering a calm state have remarkable influence on the electroencephalogram (EEG). The public health department of Wuhan Medical College discovered that there was no noticeable change of EEG in those who were asked to sit quietly for thirty minutes, but there appeared a noticeable increase of Alpha wave in those practicing still Qigong for five minutes and the increase continued during the practice for half an hour. The wave did not return to the original condition until ten minutes after the practice stopped. Elderly people had an increase of slow wave in EEG when they practiced Qigong.

The Shanghai Hypertension Research Center and Beijing Medical College also reported similar findings. A teaching panel of neuropathology in the first hospital affiliated to Shanghai First Medical College did systematic observation of EEG in twelve Qigong practitioners and found as they proceeded with their exercises that alpha wave appeared in the forehead, the wave amplitude was increasing, the cycle prolonged, and the wave was extended to the posterior; at the same time the amplitude was rising, the frequency was being slowed down but the rhythm was unchanged. (See *Shanghai Traditional Chinese Medicine* 5 [1962], p. 6.)

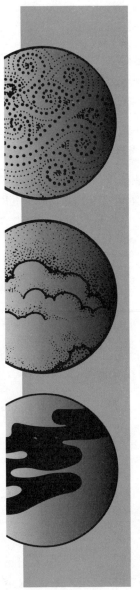

2

External Qigong

Its Origins and Development

External Qigong, which is so popular now, arose about 1978. This was after the "Gang of Four" was crushed in 1976, and after those methods of Qigong practice that had been repressed and prohibited during the Cultural Revolution were rehabilitated into society. Thereupon it spread rapidly, so that by 1978 it was quite a significant phenomenon in most large cities of the country. Caught up in the excitement were not only those who wished to use Qigong for keeping health and treating illness, but also those who wished to explain the mechanism of Qigong. Ms. Gu Hansen, a physicist and member of the Shanghai Institute of Nuclear Energy, was one of the latter group. Since 1978 she has been using her modified scientific instruments to conduct experiments on several Qigong practitioners. She published several articles describing her findings in the nationally distributed *Journal of Nature*, published in Shanghai. In these articles she stated that Qigong masters can emit several kinds of physical energy out of their body, the physical basis of which is "microwave energy," "infrared rays," "increased static electric signal," "electromagnetic waves," "weak magnetic signal," and others. (See *Journal of Nature*, vols. 6 and 10 [1979], and vol. 10 [1980].) These articles brought the term "External Qi" into general use.

Since then, some who have accepted Ms. Gu's principles have proclaimed themselves able to radiate "External Qi" after only a few days of practicing Qigong, improving their position in society considerably in the process. Because of this, "experts" in radiating "External Qi" are popping up everywhere like bamboo shoots after spring rains, all over the country.

The first use of the term "External Qi" referred to the magnetic-like signals detected after examining the Qigongists' skin with the use of measuring instruments.

During the same time period that the term and language of "External Qi" was being accepted by the general public, some Qigong masters and investigators of Qigong quickly embarked on new research, examining two aspects of the subject. First, some began to apply "External Qi" in clinical use. These people deduced that since Qigong masters could radiate physical energy, then this energy could pass through the air to the body of the patient, and therefore could adjust the condition of the patient and treat the illness. These people extended this theory, and discovered that, in some cases, even though the Qigong master was not touching the patient, he began radiating "External Energy." Some patients began experiencing heat, cold, or numbness in parts of their bodies. Some patients experienced a force pressing on their bodies, which caused them to move involuntarily. Some patients seemed to exhibit a marked improvement on the spot. This type of "External Qi" effect was not limited to one person at a time. The effects were felt by a significant number of onlookers. A number of prominent people and famous scientists became totally convinced of the effects of "External Qi" after witnessing these experiments.

The second aspect is that some persons had conducted some experiments about how External Qigong affects other materials, because they thought that if External Qigong could affect the human body, it could affect other things, too. Based on this idea, they began to do experiments on every kind of material. The numerous effects reported by them indicated that the external Qigong given out by the Qigongists could affect a variety of material, such as seeds (producing a higher germination percentage, changing the molecular structure of many substances, and making chemical reactions possible without needed temperature and pressure changes, even killing bacteria and tumor cells or causing them to grow wildly). The Qigongists radiate Qi over a short distance, or from far away (thousands of miles away). They could even dispel black clouds or cause thunderstorms to occur, rain to stop, and other phenomena. The so-called therapeutic effect and general effect on substances of Qigong have made it popular in China as well as in foreign countries.

After the proof of Qigong's effects became known, a few socially prominent people and famous scientists began to support it; and all kinds of newspapers, magazines, and radio and television stations began to get involved in spreading propaganda about Qigong. Some people who only studied Qigong for several days suddenly proclaimed themselves great masters with supernatural abilities. Those persons either traveled around the country as healers or established clinics of Qigong everywhere. Their expensive fees made them millionaires. Some became obsessed with obtaining the ability to radiate External Qigong and went around in a trancelike state all day, practicing it continually, some to the point that they became deluded or schizophrenic. Some people declared that the discovery and utilization of External Qigong was a great breakthrough in the science field of the world and that this would result in a scientific revolution.

What was the truth? Some real professional Chingongists and scientists did not follow the tide of External Qigong fanaticism or echo the views of others, and kept a sober mind. They made careful investigations and experiments and produced real scientific proof. They announced the end of fairy-tale External Qigong.

The Analysis of the Essence of the Effect of External Qigong Therapy

First, we admitted that radiating External Qigong could really have some effect on some patients or some diseases, and sometimes the effects were astonishing. However, when we explain why the effects are so remarkable, we have an explanation completely different from those who spoke in mythological terms. Those Qigongists thought that the effect was the supernatural caused by the "Qi" radiated from them. One of the most important proofs, they thought, was that patients could feel heat, cold, and tingling sensations even though the Qigongist's hands did not touch their bodies. They therefore assumed that the senses must have been stimulated by some physical function. No doubt that stimulus had to be External Qigong. Here we cannot help but state what little knowledge of psychology the Qigongists had.

Psychology regards sensation as the simplest psychological phenomenon. The senses of a human being can be divided into two types: One is internal sense and the other is external sense, including vision, hearing, smell, taste, and touch. The sense needs relevant physical stimulation to produce sensation; for example, vision needs light, hearing needs sound, smell needs odor, and the skin needs touch, pressure, or temperature stimulation.

Psychology also tells us that though all kinds of sensations can be produced by relevant physical stimulation, illusory sensations can also be produced by suggestion. Here is a famous example: A chemical professor opened a bottle on a platform and poured several drops of a solution that had no odor. He then left the platform with a distasteful expression on his face. Within a short time, the students in the front row reported a terrible odor; and gradually the students in the last row smelled it too. Psychologically, this resulted from nonphysical stimulation and suggestion brought on by the authoritative attitude and purposeful manner of the professor.

Psychology tells us that other senses can also be deceived by suggestion. For example, under hypnosis, one can drink a glass of water with keen appreciation, as though it were a soft drink. Actually, this is an illusive taste. Similarly, one can see or hear things that do not exist. (This is called "photism.") Furthermore, one can have a hallucinatory skin sensation of cold, heat, pressure, and so forth, and even experience analgesia to pain in a variety of operations. (This is called "hypnonarcosis.")

Looking at the treatment processes of External Qigong we can easily see that every Qigongist must use words, gestures, actions, eye contact, expressions, or other means to keep their patients' attention during the treatments. However, all those are just the general methods of suggestion in psychology. So we can assert categorically that there is, to some extent, suggestion in the treatment by radiating Qigong.

As to the seemingly effective treatment by external Qigong, there are three possible ways to explain the effects: First, the effect is caused by the physical External Qigong given out by the Qigongist. Second, this effect is caused by psychological suggestion in the form of Qigong. Lastly, the effect is caused by a combination of the above. Only by analyzing Qigong in this way can we get the whole answer about it. Pitifully, the Qigongists did not analyze the problem in this way. They affirmed in a nonscientific way that the effects produced by External Qigong were caused purely by physical Qigong radiation. This approach is obviously arbitrary and one-sided. If we really want to know which of the three ways mentioned above is the true cause, we must perform strict scientific research and use rigorous scientific data to prove our results.

Fortunately, this kind of experiment is not complicated; we can say it is even very simple. The main point in the experiment is to cut off any possibility of hinting or suggestion. For example, the patient can be blind-folded to prevent him from seeing when Qigong is being performed. No doubt, the subject's sensation and reaction will not be synchronous with the radiation of Qigong. If we let the Qigongist radiate Qigong quietly to the persons nearby who are unaware, no doubt, no one will feel any effect. On the contrary, let someone who has never practiced Qigong and who also cannot give out Qigong pretend to be a super-Qigongist and radiate Qigong like a real Qigongist, and quite a few persons will get the effect of the therapy on the spot. We have done these kinds of experiments repeatedly. Anyone can do it. I believe you can check any brilliant Qigongist in this manner yourself. We clearly see that Qigong does not have any effect after the suggestion is taken away. The pretender Qigongist can bring out the same effect by suggestion. So External Qigong treatment only has an effect on believers (who are easily affected by suggestion) because the treatment is featured as "if you believe, it will be effective." One who trusts science can confirm that the so-called External Qigong Effect is caused by psychological suggestion completely. If we understand External Qigong treatment from this point of view, we can understand the scientific mechanism of this therapy easily, and we can define it as a kind of suggestion therapy that uses Qigong as a stimulus replacement borrowed from Chinese national culture. Conversely, if we consider the therapeutic effect of Qigong as the result of physical External Qigong radiated by a Qigongist who has the superhuman ability to cure disease, and extend this idea, we are bound to abandon science and turn to modern superstition.

The Secret of Yan Xin's "Lectures with Qigong"

Lecturing with Qigong means that when the Qigongist is delivering a lecture to the audience, he gives out Qigong to help them at the same time. This kind of lecture caused many believers to feel a strong sense of energy, or caused them to swing a roll of their bodies involuntarily, even cry, laugh, shout. According to an investigation, the proportion of people who showed the above reactions was more than 40 percent of the attendees. Some people's diseases disappeared on the spot.

"Lectures with Qigong," during which External Qigong treatment is given along with a lecture, was a creation of Mr. Yan Xin. Yan thought that the Qigong field he radiated, combined with the the energy field of the audience, created a great power. Yan toured the country to give this kind of "Lecture with Qigong," and he declared that these performances were safe. Unfortunately, on March 7, 1990, we saw the real situation of one of these lectures from the *Xinmin Evening Paper*, which reported:

> The Shanghai auditorium, which can accommodate more than 18,000 persons, suddenly became seemingly smaller yesterday afternoon. Thousands and thousands of eyes all focused in a single direction—the rostrum. The great super-Qigongist, Yan Xin, was delivering a six-hour Qigong lecture in one session. By means of the microphone and 48 loudspeakers, his voice resounded through the whole conference hall. Yan's lecture was very smooth and steady. He talked slowly, telling the meaning of Qigong, and mentioned some diseases that can be cured. He urged the audience to keep relaxed and calm while they listened to the lecture. It was surprising that, under this condition, calm as a neighborly chat, the people in the stands could not keep still, and listeners exhibited great shows of emotion—anger, grief, or merriment.
>
> Less than five minutes into the lecture, some in the audience began

to shout, laugh, cry, and swing to and fro as if they were drunk. More and more people began to do the same. At auditorium section 20, a person about fifty years of age sang Beijing Opera at the top of his lungs. A construction worker from the railway bureau fell from his chair suddenly and rolled on the ground. Eventually his trousers were ripped and he lost his shoes. His face was flushed, and he could not say a single word. It was a long time before he calmed down. The strangest event of all happened to a young worker named Pan Jiangang, who suddenly experienced heart palpitations. His face flushed deeply, and he sweated profusely. Eventually he dared not listen any longer and ran out of the hall frightened for his life.

Many in the stands felt comfortable and not at all tired during the six-hour sitting. Certainly there were some people who did not experience any sensation during or after Yan's lecture and even suspected those people who laughed or cried were Yan's accomplices. Guo Daiwu, a thirty-year-old officer from the Industrial and Commercial Bureau of the Huangpu district in Shanghai, died suddenly while he was carefully listening to Yan's lecture. Witnesses said that after Yan's lecture began, Guo danced for joy in the stands. Eventually Guo started to spit white foam. Because the people accompanying him and the audience around him were also in a hypnotized state, they did not know such a terrible event had occurred. When someone found him, he was already dead.

Some psychological researchers conducted an investigation of several people who showed active reactions while listening to the lecture. The investigation focused on examining their receptivity to suggestion and personalities. The result indicated that the receptivity to suggestion of this group was obviously higher than that of normal people. Their personalities tended toward sensitivity. Psychologically they are childish, dependent, and immature, and they have hypochondriac and hysteric tendencies. Clearly, we can see that the behavior of the audience caused by listening to the Lecture with Qigong is the result of psychological suggestion.

An experiment that was done based on the methods of psychological suggestion further confirmed the conclusion that the effect of the Lecture with Qigong was not caused by the physical External Qigong given out by the Qigongist, but by psychological suggestion completely.

Meng Jikong, a chief leader in the Hengyang Acrobatic Troupe in the Hunan province, was not a Qigongist at all. Faced with the abuse on society perpetrated by Yan Xin's "Lectures with Qigong," he determined to conduct an experiment to expose the fraud. He propagated and touted himself as a super-Qigongist and widely advertised that he wanted to hold a Qigong meeting himself. The advertisements described a super-strong Qigong to cure disease in the meeting's lecture. More than one thousand believers attended the meeting.

After briefly covering some points needed to center attention on himself, Meng began his lecture. "Please close your eyes, straighten up your back and relax chest, keep your body relaxed, turn palms upward, and concentrate your mind on your lower abdomen [the Dantian point]. You will feel your head gradually become heavier than ever before." At this moment some began to sway to and fro. Meng Jikong went on, "Now I shall begin to give out External Qigong. Please pay attention and receive my signals. You will feel a kind of energy pushing you forward or pulling you backward. At this time, you should not resist; follow it naturally."

Then Meng began to blow into the microphone. More than 30 percent of the audience eventually began to move. "Many people have begun to move," said Meng. "Those of you who are reacting slowly, please open up and receive my signals, quickly. Relax your body; do whatever you want to. If you want to cry, you may. If you want to laugh, you may. Don't use your will to control yourself."

Thirty-five minutes later, the meeting hall boiled over. Forty percent of the audience could no longer sit calmly. Some patted their shoulders and hit themselves. Some beat their chest and stamped their feet. Some shouted loudly. Some rocked, and some rolled on the ground. Some laughed and some vomited. Some cried.

After this experiment, Mr. Meng told the truth publicly. "I am not a Qigongist, and I cannot give out External Qigong. I only caused the persons to move in my way. The way included the condition of sitting postures, and the hint and guidance of my words."

What would Mr. Yan think if he knew that Mr. Meng had repeated the same effect of a "Lecture with Qigong" without any ability to radiate Qigong? After Yan's Lecture, during which a man died, the media and public opinion became unfavorable toward him. So he went to the United

States to continue his "Lectures with Qigong." From newspaper accounts we know that many Americans, who are interested in the mysteries of the Orient, were infatuated by Yan's Lectures. However, we believe that, before long, our American friends can also regain their clear minds and see through the trick of Yan's "Lectures with Qigong."

The External Qigong Experiment Crossing National Boundaries

There are several factors contributing to the far-reaching abuse of External Qigong. Among them, the most important is that some Qigong research organizations and scientific workers produced scientific experimental proof of the existence of External Qi and its effect. All medical scientists know that, to evaluate a medical study, it is essential first not to see how remarkable the results are, but to examine the report to determine if the scientific experimental methods are reliable or not, because slight careless-ness in the methods can affect the accuracy of the experimental result directly. In real scientific studies, some results cannot pass evaluation because their methods were not reliable. There were also some real cases where pseudoscience was charged and the researchers lost their positions and reputations due to fraudulent methods. So, in evaluating an experi-mental study of External Qigong, which was declared to be a break-through in modern science, we cannot believe the results without pon-dering and checking the methods. Regretfully, in Qigong investigation few of the researchers knew medical study procedures, and trusting believers were not able to examine or determine the studies' scientific validity. Some scientists from other fields (not the Qigong field) can hardly see through the Qigong fraud because of the restriction of their knowl-edge, as if a mountain were between their specialities, even though they wanted to study Qigong. This is the current situation in Qigong study. Therefore it is the duty of professional Qigong researchers to help people recognize reliable aspects and extent of some influential experimental reports on External Qigong.

The external Qigong experiments can be roughly divided into two kinds. One is study on a physical basis of External Qigong. The representative one was what Gu Hanseng did in Shanghai. (See pages 51–52.) The other is study on External Qigong's effect. The most influential reports were those of Lida Feng from the Navy General Hospital and Lu Zuyin, Li Shengping, and Yan Xin from the Coordinated Research Group of Hsinghua University.

The experimental result showed that the physical basis of External Qigong is not credible

The fact that the experiment done by Gu Hansen proves the material basis of External Qigong is doubted by many scientists because the instrument she used was altered by herself, and the substance she thought of as the material basis of External Qigong could be checked only by herself. No one else has gotten repeat results, and the great discovery has not passed any professional evaluation so far. What is more, the colleagues who were familiar with the experiment also took a different view. Some questioned the validity of her report that infrared radiation changed before and after being subjected to radiation by Qigong. It is known that the change in a human being's skin temperature is a slow process, so it is not possible to produce an infrared modulation frequency from some tenth to tens Hz. When Gu reported she had measured the effect of the infrared radiation change while the Qigongist radiated Qigong, she demonstrated a rapidly changing state of a human's skin temperature. It means that an infrared modulation frequency at less than 10 Hz had appeared within a second. It is impossible for a human body to exhibit such a result. Unbelievably, the Qigongists did not care about scientific fact. They took Gu's experimental result as a definite scientific conclusion even though there were lots of nonscientific data. They not only believed it to be true, but also spread it among Qigong believers and quoted it in one newspaper and magazine after another. From then on, supermen with the ability of radiating External Qigong suddenly appeared all over the country one by one, with stronger and stronger Qigong. Articles about External Qigong's physical basis appeared in large numbers and more and more "miracles" occurred. Stories and excitement about these phenomena began to spread abroad.

Looking at the supposed physical basis again, we can find that Gu's examination consisted only of something with biophysical characteristics, such as sound, light, heat, magnetism, etc., which everybody experiences. In fact, the experiment on External Qigong treatment demonstrated that the patients did not show the effect of External Qigong after blocking the associated suggestion. This is enough to confirm that the effect of External Qigong was not caused by sound, light, electricity, heat, magnetism, and others. From these facts, we know that Gu's theory on the discovery of the physical basis of External Qigong was not acceptable. Ironically, the person who first found the physical basis of Qigong and was praised as the person who caused an astonishing breakthrough in Qigong study, departed from Qigong study completely and went away to focus on other subjects after some flaws in the experiment had been found. Amazingly, some external Qigongists and believers who lack knowledge of Qigong science still believe Gu's conclusion. It is a really sad and pitiful situation.

The experiment on bacteria was not repeatable

Lida Feng, a deputy chief of the Navy General Hospital, was an immunologist devoted to studying Qigong following the surge in the popularity of External Qigong. She conducted experiments on bacteria and tumor cells and gave numerous reports on experiments on External Qigong's biological effects. Taking the effect on bacteria as an example, her report said that bacteria could either be killed or proliferated by External Qigong radiated by a Qigongist with the variation of will in his mind. In order to check this result, several specialists on bacteria and researchers of the Qigong research room of the China Academy of Traditional Chinese Medicine (TCM) cooperated to undertake strict scientific research. They invited the same Qigongist who had taken part in Feng's experiment to radiate External Qigong to check the Qigong's effect on the same bacteria. Though the specialists carefully repeated the experiments several times, the fact was the same that there was no effect from the Qigong on the bacteria. The only difference between the experiments conducted by Feng and the academy was the locale and the fact the researchers were different people who obtained completely different results. Now we can only conclude that the experiment controller had processed the bacteria or altered the experimental result. This is contrary to scientific discipline. We should like to ask, do the reports on the biological effect of External Qigong and other experimental results based on this effect have much credibility? We corresponded with Feng several times and invited her to guide us in order to have a successful experiment, but she never gave us a single answer. This is typical behavior if one has something to hide. A strict scientist would never act this way.

The truth of the experiment on External Qigong at Hsinghua University

Of all the experiments on External Qigong, the most influential one known to the whole world is the experiment on changes of molecular structure by Qigong conducted by Lu Zuyin and Li Shengping in cooperation with Yan Xin in the Zigong Cooperative Research Group at Hsinghua University in 1987. This experimental result became the most authoritative scientific foundation for the validity of External Qigong, and was circulated in all kinds of media. Furthermore, the result made a tremendous impact on our society. Yan Xin himself and his experiment colleagues Lu Zuyin and Li Shengping became famous because of their experiment. Yan Xin was praised as a modern supernatural leader and invited to deliver "Lectures with Qigong." No doubt he became famous based on the reputation of Hsinghua University, to the extent many people began to criticize those who did not believe the results of the experiment. If the experiment's result was indeed what the propaganda presented, it would really have been a great breakthrough in scientific history. However, after the journalists of *Health Paper* and I began an investigation on the experiment conducted at Hsinghua University, we saw the facts were not as they claimed. The following were some serious announcements by Hsinghua University after the investigation: "They did not apply for any kind of evaluation of the study, and were not evaluated by professionals. The experiment had nothing to do with Hsinghua University, and can not be called an achievement at all":

> The University had never founded a so-called Qigong Cooperative Research Group which involved seven departments and offices, and never approved the founding of a Qigong Institute. (Refer to *Health Paper*, April 13, 1989)

Let us examine the inside information exposed by Professor Chao Nanming. In *Health Paper* 322, April 15, 1989, Chao, the head of the Biology Department, who knew of these experiments and took part in some of them, recalled: "To my knowledge, the Hsinghua Qigong Cooperative Research Group was an organization associated with the labor union of the University, founded to make Qigong popular. The university never founded a Qigong research organization which involved several departments. Two years ago, the chief head of the group, Professor Lu Zuyin, told me that Mr. Yan Xin wanted to do some experiments at Hsinghua University, and Professor Lu hoped I would cooperate with him. I agreed, subject to two requirements. One was that the course of the experiment should be designed by us, and the sample and the preparation should be made by us also. The other was that only with our agreement could any report be published. After Yan arrived, we undertook experiments on the change of liquid crystal phase, and the ultraviolet spectra change on DNA from bovine thymus. The whole process was relatively rough at that time. There was no temperature-control system and no standard temperature curve. The experiment was done completely by Yan Xin himself and repeated only three times. In the study on Qigong, I thought it should progress from simple to complex experiments, in order to see whether Qigong can affect molecular structure, and then see the effects on animal cells and then human cells. Later Lu consulted with Li Shengping (a Lecturer in the Chemistry Department at the university, the deputy head of the group) about doing experiments using Raman laser. In fact Lu and Li had never studied the Raman laser. They asked one of my postgraduates to do this experiment with Yan. After the experiment, the postgraduate said that the experiment was not accurate. According to common international protocol, academic articles published in a journal should involve blind-control experiments, strict design, and repeatability. So when Lu asked me whether the series of experimental studies on Qigong could be published, I said that it is too early to reach a conclusion at present. The thing was that Lu and Li combined three articles into one and published it while I was away on official business without my permission. What is more, they recorded the effect of External Qigong at a long distance (more than six kilometers) in the article. I was very angry when I learned what they had done and criticized them for their careless attitude.

Later Lu gave a report about ultraviolet absorption of bovine thymus DNA in the name of the Qigong Cooperative Research Group of Hsinghua University (at that time, he had already left the university) at a national Qigong conference. *Guangming Daily* published that on the first page as important news. Li argued with Lu over who would be the paper's first author, then Li was interviewed by a journalist from the *Chinese Youth* newspaper in the name of the group, and that newspaper published Li's article on the front page."

Also Li was interviewed by some relevant leaders and so he became popular in our country. Concerned about this matter, in September 1987 my department had written a report to the Scientific Research Office and the Party Committee of the university to clarify the case. However, Li did not pay any attention to this. Thereafter, he published Qigong research papers in a variety of national and international journals numerous times. Among them, the most influential one was the paper entitled "Experimental Research on the External Qigong Effect on Substances Over a Distance of 2,000 Kilometers." As to whether External Qigong can change molecular structure when the Qigongist is 2,000 kilometers away, you can easily make a judgment from general scientific knowledge. In this experiment, there were at least two doubtful points. First is that the temperature accuracy in the article was 0.01 degrees, which is impossible to measure at Hsinghua University. Also, the report did not give the standard error. Second is that the samples in the control and experimental group were only 100 meters apart. Even using a laser, one would have difficulty finding the true mark. Even if the experiment had been scientific, and even if it had been a great discovery, more thorough and more repeatable experiments are in order. Besides these concerns, our investigation indicated that they did not adhere to scientific procedures in the experiment: They neglected to strictly control the water samples; theirs were obtained from different running water sources. Because the running water sources were different, how could they say the change was caused by External Qigong?

The myth that External Qigong could change the molecular structure of substances by Yan's and other Qigongists' Qigong was absolutely unveiled. Does such a report on External Qigong deserve our respect? Shouldn't those people who believed and spread the report get the whole truth and the facts?

The truth of the experimental report given by Zhang Xiangyu

Zhang Xiangyu, another quite influential Qigongist, has become famous in recent years. She declared that her Qigong was natural and that she was a supernatural being. She propagated the idea that her Qigong had passed examination and experimental study. Her "experimental report" made many people, even some scientists, trust her. Let us see what the inside story of this so-called scientific experiment really is.

Like many other Qigongists, Zhang went to Wuhan University, Tongji Medical University, and other institutions to conduct some experiments through the channel of her connections. It was not the case that these universities invited her to do the study. More importantly, the result of the experiments was not reliable.

Professor Bi, of the Microbiology Institute of Tongji Medical University, had taken part in the experiment. She explains, "The experiment was not complete, because of the few attempts and no repeatability. Most of the results of the experiment were recorded only one time by us, so we never gave any conclusive report on it. We only wanted to accumulate data to further the subject of Qigong study, and wrote a report of the results. Strictly speaking, this was only a record of the experimental process."

Professor Bi remembered that in the experiments with Zhang and others, the subjects of inquiry included the effect of Qigong on the phagocytic function of macrophages from mouse abdominal cavity fluid, on the change of white cells in blood, on the serum titer of hepatitis B surface antigen in hepatitis patients, on the lymphocyte surface antigen in the extracorporeal blood, and other experiments. Ironically, only experiments on the life expectancy of the mouse with a heart transplant got a relatively "reliable" experimental effect. The mouse in the experimental group lived longer than that in the control group. But it could not be repeated. Therefore, there was no way to determine whether the Qigong radiated by Zhang and her students affected the life span of the mouse with a transplanted heart. As to how Zhang procured a record of the experiment, Professor Bi recalled, "After the experiments, Zhang did not come back to Tongji Medical University again. Her students waited for the results at the university. Generally speaking, we don't give the experimental results to the Qigongists themselves. However, they inquired about the results repeatedly, and said they would take the experimental results to Beijing and report it to the leaders of the Qigong Science Institute of China. Our researchers had to give them a copy by writing it on common letter paper."

Professor Bi was very angry when, unexpectedly, they published this experimental material in the name of the Microbiology Department at Tongji Medical University without the consent of the University and the researchers. She said, "Zhang's experimental research report, linked with the Microbiology Institute of Tongji Medical University, published in the book *Great Nature Soul*, shouldn't be taken as a conclusion of the experiment."

Another chief participant in the study was Professor Li from the Examination Center of Wuhan University. Professor Li said straightforwardly that it was an experiment with a short time of preparation, an imperfect experimental design, bad cooperation between Zhang and the researchers, and with a fraudulent evaluation of the results.

Like Tongji Medical University, Wuhan University took few samples in experiments. All subjects tested were only tested one time without any repeated examination. The report was only a result report on single experiments.

During the experiments, examiners knew that the samples had not changed, but they (Zhang and her students) shouted "It has changed!" loudly, and said only people who possessed a special Qigong vision that allowed them to see what common people cannot, could perceive this change.

This is the truth about the scientific experiments. (Refer to *Health Paper*, July 28, 1990.)

Science is a strict, honest matter. It does not allow any trickery. The facts will show those people who casually come to conclusions with good intentions but wrong scientific design, that their conclusions are wrong. The history of Qigong development will also record the disgraceful story of those who only wanted to gain fame and profit for themselves by spreading Qigong in a fraudulent way and thus cause the reputation and development of Qigong to suffer a heavy loss.

The Recognition of the Essence of Qigong

One should be able to define each new scientific subject in a few words that are easily understood by nonprofessionals; thus general knowledge (properties, characteristics, and actions) about the subject can be easily accepted. However, Qigong science is different from any other subject. Besides religion, Qigong claims more believers than any other subject. Ironically, if we asked believers what Qigong is, we would get various answers. Most people only know Qigong dimly, and cannot explain it clearly or concisely. Even the Qigong research professionals themselves cannot give a clear definition. Often they give Qigong many definitions. Among them there is one common point; namely, they all think practicing Qigong is a way to cultivate essential (or primary) Qi (energy). Those who have been nurtured in traditional Chinese culture perhaps can roughly understand what to cultivate essential Qi means. To Westerners (Americans and Europeans) it is another confusing story.

Logic tells us that a definition is the logical way to expose the essence of a concept; that is, to find with simple but clear words the essential nature of the subject that the concept encompasses. So determining the essential nature of Qigong is the premise for clarification of the definition and concept of Qigong.

It is known that the essential nature is that which makes something unique and distinguished from others. The essential nature is the dominant and determinant position among all aspects of a subject. In that way, which aspect occupies this position among all aspects of Qigong?

First, let's look over some statements given by the ancient Chinese. There is an early classic book on treating disease called *The Yellow Emperor's Internal Classic*, written more than 2,000 years ago, which recorded abundant statements in the first chapter on the essential nature of Qigong. For example, "The heart is the Emperor, and controls mental activity. If the 'Emperor' is sensible, the subordinates (other organs) will be in order. Preserved in this way, one will have a long life. If the Emperor is not sensible, other organs will be in trouble. Continuing in this way, one's health will be bad." (In this case, they mean the general attitude or intent of a person.) This statement definitely points out the importance of mental activity in the process of preserving one's health. The phrases "Without distracting thought, genuine Qi will be in the body and a sound mind will be preserved; how can you suffer?" "Keeping a sound mind independently," "Calm down your mind without distracting thoughts," and others further set forth the idea that entering a special calm state by adjusting one's mental activity (psychological activity) is the crucial point of Qigong practice. The book *Prescriptions Worth a Thousand Pieces of Gold for Emergencies*, written by Sun Simiao, the famous TCM doctor in the Tang dynasty, recorded, "Think with your eyes closed; imagine that you can see a current of wonderful primordial Qi in the sky like a purple cloud, forming an umbrella over you with five colors. Then this Qi descends to the hair and slowly enters your body through the top of your head, just like when the sun comes out after rain and the clouds melt into a mountain. The Qi penetrates into skin and muscle, and gradually goes down into the abdomen. At last the extremities and five organs all get nurtured as water penetrating into the ground. When it penetrates thoroughly you will perceive a gurgling sound from the abdomen. Keep your mind and thought focused. Don't relax them too soon. The Qi will soon go into the Yongquan point." This statement illustrates that the process of a Qigong exercise is actually a course of adjusting mental activity. It is a self-adjusting psychological activity process that focuses on self-suggestion, and includes imagination, self-sensation, concentration, and attention on the self. The wonderful primordial Qi and its flow on this course is entirely the result of self-suggestion using one's own imagination as one of the components. Looking casually into any one of the ancient books about Qigong practice, we will find all the contents similar. It is our conclusion that the essential nature of Qigong is a course of adjusting mental psychological activity.

Certainly, nowadays Qigong exercises include three elements: adjustment of the mind, breath, and body. However, adjustment of the mind has the dominant role in Qigong practice. Though in some ancient and current Qigong methods, such as the method of exhaling and inhaling, the Qi-circulating methods, the Qi swallowing methods, the way of breathing has been especially emphasized, the aim of all the methods and exercises is to let Qigong practitioners concentrate their attention on breath, which is really a way to help them calm down, and replace millions of evanescent thoughts with one idea during the breathing. Similarly, though gestures and movements may be stressed in some Qigong exercises, the movements actually serve as special suggestions used for the adjustment of mind, such as embracing a globe, holding the moon with two hands, and holding the air in the hands. Thus it is obvious that breathing and movements in Qigong practice indeed are the ways to assist the practitioners to adjust the mind. Another fact accepted in Qigong circles can also confirm this: During the process of Qigong practice, there may be no special demands on movement, such as in the motionless Qigong practice; or no special demands on one's way of breathing, such as in the natural breath Qigong practice. However, any Qigong practice must include the adjustment of the mind. In short, it may be called Qigong practice without adjusting one's breathing and body, but it cannot be called Qigong practice without adjusting the mind. "Practicing Qigong depends on the mind absolutely" is an accurate summary of the main idea of Qigong practice in ancient times.

Based on the ancient and current Qigong theories and actual Qigong exercises, we can easily make the judgment that Qigong is a method of keeping fit that takes the theory of adjusting the mind in TCM as its core principle. In modern words, Qigong can be defined as a kind of psychosomatic exercise method whose essence is self-suggestion, which can bring the mind into an autohypnotic state. That is the so-called calm state in Qigong practice by means of self-adjustment of the psychological/physiological/morphological reaction link so as to prevent and cure disease.

The course of Qigong practice is a process whereby people learn healthful behavior and which is fixed by means of conditioned reflex. Also so-called External Qigong therapy only helps patients through suggestion, which causes a change due to a psychological/physiological/morphological reaction link in the patients.

Originally, the essential character of Qigong, which is adjusting the mind through practice, has already demonstrated that Qigong is a subject that involved the concrete application and development of the theory of mind adjustment and emotional conditions in TCM. Unfortunately, a general phenomenon occurring in present Qigong circles obliterates this character. The means of adjusting mind is applied during instruction, learning, and practice, even while radiating Qigong, but when discussing

Qigong concept and theory, the Qigongists often obstinately refer the essential character of Qigong to cultivating the essential primordial Qi, so produce a contradiction between the practice and theory. In order to clarify the cause of the contradiction, it is necessary to recall the changing course of the selection and intention of the Qigong concept.

Though the word "Qigong" can be found in some ancient books, it did not have the current meaning until the establishment of new (post-revolutionary) China. Some called the practice of health preservation which stressed the method of breathing Qigong therapy, but this was not prevalent in the whole country at that time. In 1955 the clinical work of the Qigong Experimental Group in Tangshan, headed by Liu Guizheng, was praised by the National Health Department, which propagated the event to the whole country by broadcasts and press releases. And the first professional office of Qigong in the country, the Tangshan Qigong Sanitarium, was set up. Later, with the support of the government, the Beidaihe Qigong Sanatorium was set up. Liu Guizheng became famous and a figure of authority because of the timeliness of his research and topographical advantage. People from all over the country came to learn Qigong. He went everywhere to deliver lectures on Qigong, and even stayed at the national central government residences for a long time and taught Qigong to top leaders, including the former chairman of the country. Led by Liu, not only was Qigong therapy spread widely throughout the whole country, also the expression "Qigong therapy," which was selected by Liu Guizheng, referring to ideas of his predecessors, disseminated extensively in the country. Thus the word "Qigong" evolved.

The history of the spread of Qigong therapy can be verified, but there were some contradictions between the former and later explanations given by Liu. In the book *Qigong Therapy Practice*, published in September 1957, he wrote, "Why do we call this Qigong therapy? 'Qi' means breath here, and 'gong' is the practice of continually adjusting breath and movement. Qigong therapy, reformed and studied from a medical viewpoint, is used to treat diseases and preserve health without formerly associated superstition." In that statement, and what he explained in the book about the breathing exercise which he gained from a peasant in Hebei Province, we can clearly see that Liu regarded breathing adjustment as the essential character of Qigong at that time. This changed the original meaning of the

Qigong concept, with the emphasis on adjusting the mind, which had lasted for several thousand years.

Some clearheaded scholars in the Qigong circle raised an objection to the selection and definition of the word "Qigong" from the very beginning. For example, Mr. Jiang Weiqiao, a famous Qigong expert in Shanghai, said in his book *Discussing Qigong Therapy*, "Now everyone calls it Qigong; actually this name is not suitable. Because 'Qigong' has already become popular, I have to use this name. In fact it was called the 'healthy living' method in ancient times." In the article entitled "Some Experiences with Qigong Therapy," Mr. Li Lizhi pointed out, "There are always some people who understand Qigong as practicing Qi (breath) just as the name implies. So they pay a great deal of attention to the word 'Chi' only. Thus a lot of corrupt practices appeared." The situation that Mr. Li was afraid of has now become reality: Many believers have gone crazy practicing Qigong.

The regrettable thing is that facing divergent views, Liu did not get a clear picture and went further with this wrong idea. In the preface of the book *Qigong Therapy Practice* (second edition, June 1982), he said, "According to the classic theory, we called this method, which mainly cultivates the vital Qi, Qigong. We consider that the Qi in Qigong practice not only includes the Qi in breathing but also the vital Qi in the body." In the first paragraph of the same book he wrote, "We called the body-strengthening method of cultivating primordial Qi as Qigong. This sufficiently reflects the view of TCM theory that takes the Qi as the foundation of the body." In the third paragraph of the book he wrote, "The Qi in Qigong practice mainly refers to genuine (primary) Qi." Thus it is clear that the contents of the Qigong concept as defined by Liu got a substantive change. The change in cognition from the breathing Qi to the vital Qi inside the body was a result of the change in thought. (In fact, this cognition transfer from the literal meaning of Qigong was presented not only by Liu at that time.) The transfer deviated from the essential character of Qigong: adjusting mind and focusing thought obscured the essential concept of Qigong. It further established the theoretical foundation for some who changed the view of inner Qi to the view of radiating Qigong from the inside. It was also the theoretical source of the current phenomena such as the appearance of "External Qigong supermen," reports of all kinds of External Qigong miracles, and Qigong becoming deified and commercialized.

To sum up, changes in the explanation of the intention of Qigong and the change in the concept of the content of Qi, which have gone in three steps: from the breathing Qi, to internal Qi, then to the radiation of Qi (Qigong), entirely deviated from the essential character of Qigong. With the aid of the media blitz involving newspapers, radio stations, TV stations, which added fuel to the flame, External Qigong became a kind of culture that strongly affected people or a kind of social ideology, almost a religion, with it as the object of adoration by the belivers in the Qigong circle. The theoretical system of External Qigong was founded on the basis of illusion. The system actually was the theoretical basis of pseudo-Qigong and Qigong chaos.

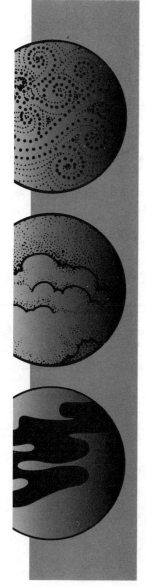

3

Itinerant Quackery and Qigong

The meaning of the term *quackery* is complex, and is seldom qualified in modern Chinese language. Referring to people, the term covers two groups: (1) forces that are beyond the power of government. Some of these developed into sinister gangs, such as the notorious Qinhong Gang, Tongshan Society, and another reactionary secret society named "Yiguandao Religion," which, under the cover of religious activities, served Japanese invaders and Kuomintang reactionaries in old China. (2) Traveling artists who earned their living through quack skills and arts. There were eight types of such business people, including fortune-tellers, drug sellers, acrobatic performers, singers, and con artists.

Special behaviors, jargon, and relations existed in the quack community. Quack societies followed a common rule in relations with outsiders —to maintain their scam despite the differences and contradictions that existed among themselves.

What is the scam?

The key to the scam is the secret through which quacks defrauded people out of their money. They would rather lose a bar of gold than to reveal this secret. Simply, all the scam methods, or the key points of quack practices, have been borrowed by some Qigong "experts" and labeled as "science."

It is no exaggeration that nearly 99.99 percent of all the "kung fu" performed in the manner of Qigong are tricks. Quackery was always part of traditional culture but not a desirable part of it. There is wit, cunning, and cleverness within quackery, and therefore it is necessary and beneficial to examine it.

Some false Qigong experts have cheated a large number of people, including some famous scientists, through their so-called Chundian Method. There is nothing in common between such quack practices and our real Qigong studies.

Former quack practices have become the super "kung fu" of today's false Qigong experts. This is abnormal and an affront to human civilization.

Having studied Qigong for many years, I have a great interest in magic, acrobatics, psychology, hypnotism, and medicine. I have myself practiced Qigong, but I don't want to bring disgrace to Qigong by claiming the title of Qigong expert. I would feel ashamed to make money from it.

In August 1990 I exposed the secrets of a dozen so-called Qigong performances before members of the press, medicine, and sciences. In September I collaborated with Professor Guo Zhengyi, of the Chinese Academy of Sciences, in filming a television program called "The Secrets of Qigong Experts" in which I demonstrated and exposed the secrets of over thirty popular special kung fu Qigong in the country. This program has been seen both at home and abroad. In October my first book (as co-author) was published. Then in December I gave three lectures on Qigong at Beijing University in which I disputed the conclusions of some other Qigong scholars and provoked a good deal of attention.

Later, in May 1991, I was invited to perform and give lectures at several prominent universities in Shanghai. After this successful academic trip, I was also invited to tour several other cities around the country. It was also in May 1991 that my second book, *Exposing Secrets of False Qigong*, rolled off the press.

Five months later I was invited by CCTV to help create a television series called *Sudden Enlightenment*, in which I demonstrated false Qigong through physical, chemical, and psychological principles. In January 1993 my third book, *To Tell Falsity Among Qigong Practices*, was published by the Publishing House of Overseas Chinese. Then in February I offered an invitation through the monthly magazine *Law and Life* for the popular "Qigong" expert Zhang Baoshen to receive a strict scientific examination before an audience.

The reason for my activities is that I have realized my responsibility to tell the world the truth since I am an expert. There is an old Chinese saying that "Amateurs look for enjoyment while experts look for principles." I hope that all people will look for the methods of false Qigong practices.

The Truth of Magic Tricks of Pseudo-Qigong*

One-Finger "Tough Qigong"

It was reported in the *China Youth Daily* that a young man stopped an electric fan by putting his finger between the blades. The young man was demonstrating what is called *Yizhichan*, a kind of tough Qigong. His show shocked many people who dared not try this stunt lest their fingers be cut off.

Is it necessarily true that fingers will be hurt by an electric fan? If you are interested, I'll tell you a secret.

1. Any electric fan can be used, no matter what brand it is.

2. If one is afraid of being hurt, the stronger middle finger or index finger, or both can be used (but that will not be called *Yizhichan*, but *Erzhichan*, meaning two-finger Qigong).

3. The front safety grid is opened.

4. The fan is plugged in and turned on at the lowest speed.

5. The finger is inserted into the rotating blades firmly. The only thing required at this moment is courage.

---

*See disclaimer on page 12. *Do not attempt these tricks yourself.*

There is nothing behind this but a little trick. The finger will first touch the slope of the blades and there is no danger of its being cut off.

Lifting a Bicycle with the Mouth

A group of acrobats, Wushu, and Qigong performers came to the newly opened business center in Xidan, Beijing, in 1989. One of the performances they put on was lifting a bicycle with the mouth. A handsome young man in a splendid costume walked onto the stage accompanied by music. A black bicycle was also pushed onto the stage. Standing at the rear of the bicycle, he tied a towel to the luggage carrier. Then he put his hands on his hips and put the towel in his mouth. With a sudden jerk, he lifted the bicycle. He pulled the bicycle around to thunderous applause.

"How long did it take you to acquire this ability?" I asked him afterward.

"About a dozen years. People have different qualifications."

One day, a year later, I walked out of my room and suddenly had an idea at the sight of my bicycle. I found a towel and tied it to the bicycle, bent down, put the towel in my mouth, and tried hard to lift it—and I succeeded. I was excited but, at the same time, felt angry that I had been deceived. Any man can do this!

Lifting Objects with Unseen Force

At the 1988 CCTV spring festival party, superman Zhang Jialing from Hubei lifted a basin using his "thought." The TV audience will perhaps remember that Zhang Jialing, dressed as a warrior, went onstage with an amiable smile. After some exaggerated movements, he put his right hand into an empty basin and, as the TV audience saw, lifted it without difficulty. Zhang Jialing has been well known ever since, and his martial arts school has been crowded with students and worshipers.

What was in Zhang Jialing's hand? How did he lift the basin?

If your sewer is jammed, you will probably need a plunger, which is usually available in hardware stores. This device inspired Zhang Jialing's performance. But his tool was much smaller, a kind of clothes hook with a rubber suction cup. A thin wire or thread may be substituted for the hook. The idea is to fasten the suction cup onto the hand. The cost will be less than one yuan.

Damaging Objects with Thought

A master took off his coat and began to move about the house. Then he asked three old men to hang a banana on a tree which was about one hundred meters away. He then quickened his pace and breathed heavily, and suddenly shouted two loud, short cries while fiercely waving his hand twice in the direction of the banana. He then gradually became quiet. His hands moved down to the front of his belly, finishing his performance.

He said quietly, "Please peel the banana and see what happened."

The crowd came closer and saw that the banana had been cut into three parts.

The banana had actually been prepared before the performance. To do this, pierce the banana with a needle and carefully swerve the needle back and forth horizontally, taking care not to damage the peel. The banana will be cut but the outside peel will appear untouched.

Hammering Head

This performance is quite popular. A master puts four to six bricks on top of his head, and an assistant hits the bricks with a large hammer. Usually the bricks are smashed while the master is not hurt at all.

If you are interested in how this is done, you can observe a working bricklayer. With a cleaver, he can cut a brick held in his hand into any shape without hurting his hand.

Generally, only a bit of a shock is felt when the brick breaks. It can be tried on the feet and legs. A brick is placed on the head, not directly on the Baihui acupuncture point which is on the top of the skull. It is better to put it near the forehead. The brick is held with the left hand, and hit with a hammer lightly. The brick breaks before the vibration can be felt. Now it's time for an assistant to hammer the brick.

Qigong masters can withstand more intense vibration than untrained people simply because they have gotten used to it through practice. The same holds true for other exercises. American boxers can deliver much more forceful strikes not because of their knowledge of Qigong but because of their intensive practice.

Why will the skull not be hurt if a brick is put between it and a hammer? If you throw a small ball forcefully at an orange, you will find that the orange will not be knocked away; the same principle applies to the performance of hammering the head. Getting an object to move is determined by force as well as time. When the hammer hits the brick, the brick will usually break before the force is entirely transmitted to the skull. This is a basic principle of physics. So the assistants must be quick and not strike too hard.

Breaking Stone on One's Belly

The performer usually lies down on his back. Some lie suspended between two benches. Several young men put a large stone on his belly. An assistant will swing an eighteen-pound sledgehammer and smash the stone without hurting the performer. The audience is excited at the scene but find it difficult to understand why the human body remains intact after the large, hard stone is broken.

In fact, the performance has nothing to do with Qigong. Some acrobats in the old days made their living doing the same stunt. They labeled it a secret of their heritage. Recently, some swindlers began calling it a kind of "tough Qigong," since Qigong is becoming more and more popular.

The crux of the performance is:

1. *The choice of stones.* Not all stones can be broken this way. There is a kind of stone in north China that will remain intact no matter how hard it's struck with an eighteen-pound hammer. The performers will be unlucky if they use this kind of stone. To guarantee success, the stone must be brittle and about 10 cm thick. Its weight should be under 150 kg. Soft and cracked stones will not do. According to experience, tombstones are the best for the performance.

2. *The manner of striking the stone.* The assistant must strike with considerable force, but he must be quick. He must exaggerate his movements. The audience will usually be convinced that he has spared no effort.

3. *What the performer must do.* When the hammer comes down, he must stick his chest out until the hammer hits the stone.

The principle here is the same as hammering the head. The stone has been broken before the force is transmitted onto the body. An old acrobat said she used to do this in the old days. Seeing that she is so thin and small, I don't think she was strong when she was young. "How could you manage with such a large stone?" I asked. "Did you know Qigong?"

"No. I had never heard of it."

Holding Back a Motorcycle

A motorcycle was started, and the driver was ready to charge forward. The performer tied a towel onto the back of the motorcycle and took the other end of the towel in his mouth. He then gestured to the driver to go ahead. The motorcycle charged several times, and soon was at full throttle, but could move only a little. The audience could see that the performer was making a great effort to hold the motorcycle back. The motorcycle was eventually pulled back for five or six meters. The wonderful performance won thunderous applause. The audience could see that one end of the towel had been stained with blood.

What the audience didn't know is that any strong young man can do the same. A light motorcycle has a force of 20 kg when it is in third gear. And everybody knows that it doesn't take a 60 kg force to pull a 60 kg man.

Four points must be remembered:

1. The performer bites the towel fully, using every tooth, and doesn't give up even if there is a risk of being pulled down.

2. The first gear is the most powerful. The motorcycle can be put into second or even third gear. There will not be any problems.

3. The performer doesn't do this with any people other than his partners, and doesn't use any motorcycle other than the one with which he is accustomed.

4. The performer does some exercises before performing. He makes his joints, spine, and especially cervical vertebrae as flexible as possible.

Generally speaking, good health, courage, and *care* are the most important ingredients. You don't have to know Qigong. A half-hour exercise is enough.

Some performers will say that this is a secret passed down from their ancestors, but chances are that there were motorcycles in those times.

Holding Back a Truck

A truck was inching forward while a Qigong master was trying to pull it back. Eventually the truck stopped. The master was visibly making a greater effort, and the truck did seem to be at full throttle. The audience was astonished to see that the truck was being pulled back toward the Qigong master.

The secret was that the driver was an accomplice. When the master was ready, the driver opened throttle and the truck started to move. The master had no way to stop the truck at this time. The driver then took the truck out of gear, and so the truck would not move no matter how hard the driver pushed the throttle. So long as the brakes were not on, the master could easily get the truck to move.

Knocking a Tombstone Apart with the Head

This is a typical "kung fu" stunt. Most performers have trained for a fairly long time, but only a kind of stamina training. They first hit their heads with planks, and then with bricks and sandbags. This training actually has nothing to do with Qigong. After a period of training, anybody can endure the shock. The performers mentioned so far have at least spent some time training. But some swindlers today also proclaim themselves "tough Qigong" masters. Stonemasons know their secrets.

One day I went to a place where tombstones are produced. The people there looked at me scornfully when I said that I wanted a tombstone for a Qigong performance. They had been acquainted with many Qigong masters, including a very famous one who was the hero of the film *Chinese Tough Qigong*. These "masters" looked for soft and rotten stones, broke them, and then put them back together with glue. Thus was a tombstone made ready for a "tough Qigong" performance. The masons believe that there are some people who can break some stones with their heads. It depends on the structure of the material.

An expert told me another secret. During a performance, a piece of iron is usually put behind the tombstone. When the stone is hit, it will break beginning at the part that strikes against the iron.

Swallowing Glass

A Qigong master broke a ceramic bowl and asked the audience to see whether it was authentic. Then the master moved around and muttered to himself. He picked up a fragment of the ceramic bowl, put it into his mouth, and began to chew. After a while, he opened his mouth and let the audience have a look at the ground ceramic. Then he drank some water and swallowed the ceramic with difficulty. When he opened his mouth again, the ceramic disappeared.

There is another kind of performance. In this, the performer swallows the ceramic without biting. And some of them eat electric bulbs and glass. The audience will feel that it's too awful and sometimes will suggest one not perform this anymore. But the master would say that it's no more difficult than biting sunflower seeds. He would say he had been trained for many years.

What the performers eat is not ceramic but a kind of ready-made substitute that looks like ceramic but is much crisper. Quack remedy sellers in the old days would shout that their remedies could dissolve ceramics. They put a piece of ceramic substitute into their poultices and secretly pinched it to crush it. Buyers and onlookers would believe them. Though the old-time performers did this frequently, there have never been any known casualties. However, swallowing something like this is not comfortable; it requires great courage. Courage is not Qigong. Swindlers will be despised by more and more people when their secret is known.

Boring a Brick with a Finger

Many Qigong masters like to give this performance, for it is welcomed by the audience. Is it that easy? Some of the best soldiers from the Beijing Armed Police Qigong team tried very hard but failed. They eventually bored a hole in a brick with a steel drill.

There are two ways that the so-called boring a brick with a finger trick is performed.

1. *Covering up*: A hole is bored in a brick in advance and this brick is put among ordinary bricks. It is important that the performer knows

where it is and the audience should be allowed to come near it. The performer pretends to pick up a brick at random and lets the audience see only one side. And then he begins to bore the other side.

2. *Casting*: A hole is bored in a brick in advance. It isn't drilled through. Some brick powder is put into the hole which is sealed with a mixture of egg white, millet gruel, and starch, or just with mud. The rest is easy.

Breaking a Brick with a Glass Cup

"Please look at the cup," said the performer who was on stage with a glass cup in his hand. "I'm going to break the brick on the ground with this ordinary cup." The performer exercised for a while, then struck the brick with the cup. The red brick was broken, and the cup was intact. He continued pounding the brick with the cup until the brick was smashed. Three points should be made:

1. The brick is hit with the bottom of the cup only, for it is more solid than the other parts.

2. There is an angle of 70 to 80 degrees between the bottom of the cup and the surface of the brick. That is, the brick is hit only with the rim of the bottom.

3. Knock away from the edge of the brick.

It is not difficult to perform this trick. The initial exercise is only to deceive the audience.

Stroking a Red-hot Iron Bar

A one-inch-thick iron bar was taken out of the fire, and its color immediately turned from white to dark red, with some sparks flying about. Holding the iron bar with a pair of tongs with his right hand, a Qigong master stared at it for a while, and then stroked his forehead with his left hand as if he were making up his mind. He shouted suddenly and stroked the red-hot bar quickly. The audience heard something burning and saw a wisp of smoke. The master switched the tongs to his left hand and repeated the movement with his right hand. The audience could smell that something had been burned. The Qigong master showed his hands to the audience. People found that there were no injuries except some dark colors.

This performance is actually the easiest. An iron bar can be heated red-hot above 800 degrees centigrade. To heat it white requires 1,000 degrees. When the iron is red-hot, the performer quickly strokes it with his right hand and nothing will happen. To make the burning sound and white smoke, he applies some petroleum jelly to his forehead. He strokes his forehead before stroking the iron. It is the petroleum jelly that burns. The burning sound and the white smoke makes him a hero.

How can an ordinary person stroke a red-hot iron? Only some cells of the hand can feel heat and transmit it to the brain through nerves. The larger the area exposed to heat, the more heat a person will feel. We can touch a boiling kettle quickly, but cannot put our hands into the boiling water. Some people can dip their hands into boiling water only because there is a layer of keratose (callus) on their palms. Though the iron is hot, it is still bearable if stroked as quickly as possible, for the hand leaves the bar before the performer can feel it. And the keratose layer on the palm is usually thicker than in most places on the body, and this helps one endure the heat.

Being Immune from an Ax

This is a standard in the repertoire of many Qigong troupes and has a long history. After taking some deep breaths, the master picks up a sharp ax and cuts some wood as a demonstration that the ax is real. (Some masters cut some tree twigs, turnips, and so forth.) Then he takes off his shirt and exposes his strong, masculine body. He bravely slices at his puffed-out chest. The audience finds that the master is not injured at all!

How can the master endure this punishment with such a heavy ax? The tip of the ax that is used to cut the twigs is sharp, but the lower section is blunt, and this is the part that he uses to strike his chest.

Eating Burning Coal

An old man took out a piece of red charcoal from a stove with a pair of chopsticks, put it into his mouth, and began to chew on it. Soon his teeth and lips turned black. He then went on to chew several more pieces.

The charcoal used is made of the lightest wood, and is therefore soft and crisp. To make it, a kind of wood is put into a fire, and when it turns red, it is put into cold water.

The charcoal is red when taken out of the stove, but the core is still black. The sparks actually come from the bamboo chopsticks. When put into the mouth, the performer feels it burning, but this doesn't last. Chewing it is not overly painful as the core is still damp and black. Chewing the second piece is much easier, since the mouth has been protected by the damp residue of the previous piece.

Eating Fire

This is another performance that has been presented by CCTV. The Qigong master held an iron bar with some cotton bound to one end of it. He dipped the cotton into some gasoline and then lit a fire. Holding the iron with his right hand, the master blew on it and the fire burned brightly.

Calmly, the master posed and slowly raised the fire. Staring at the fire for a while, he suddenly waved the iron, and some sparks flew out. Again holding the iron steadily, he squatted and opened his mouth. He slowly put the fire into his mouth and kept it there for about ten seconds! When he at last removed the iron, he opened his mouth, and the audience was surprised to see that he was not burned at all.

This is not Qigong; it does not even have anything to do with skill.

The cotton was dipped not into gasoline, but into kerosene. These two fuels are quite different. When gasoline is lit it flares out in all directions, whereas a kerosene fire burns mostly upward. When the burning cotton is put in the middle of the mouth, with the head pointed upward, nothing will happen. To ensure that no superfluous burning kerosene drops into his mouth, the performer must shake the iron bar forcefully. An inexperienced performer might repeat the shaking maneuver for safety. Also, while doing this stunt, the performer must summon more saliva in his mouth as another protective measure. Performers among local folks sometimes keep some water that has been used to cook the rind of pomegranates in their mouths, but this is usually unnecessary.

Standing on a Balloon

Again at the CCTV's "Spring Festival Evening Party," Zhang Jialing's "light" Qigong impressed the audience. He went out on stage, carrying several big balloons. He put two balloons on the ground and laid a piece of plywood on top of them. He drew a deep breath and stepped onto the plywood. The two balloons supported a strong man's weight! The home audience was overwhelmed.

This trick works best with balloons with a diameter of 15 to 25 cm. One balloon is put inside the other, and a little air is blown into it. This process is repeated. Once the performer is atop the balloons, he can keep his balance. He could even stand on one balloon.

Standing on a Matchbox

This is another popular "light" Qigong performance. During the performance, the master has no way of making himself light, but only tries to keep his balance. In other words, this has nothing to do with Qigong, but is a kind of skill.

The matchboxes used for this performance are different from ordinary ones. It is impossible for the audience to notice this difference from a distance. They see that the matchboxes are empty, but they do not see that thin steel sheets have been inserted into them. The performers have to be quick to hide the special matchbox if someone from the audience wants to check it closely.

Hanging onto a Fluorescent Tube

This performance became popular after being presented on CCTV's "Spring Festival Evening Party." A fluorescent tube is made of glass and is, of course, fragile. What's more, the tube is dangling on a pair of paper rings. How can it hold a man's weight? The bewildered audience naturally attributes it to Qigong.

Now let me tell you how it works. Two paper rings are placed on an iron rod or a wooden stick that is firmly fixed to the ceiling. The paper is actually a special cardboard of unusual strength. I found a piece of this material at one performance and couldn't tear it apart until I found someone to help me. The ends of the two "paper" rings should be well glued.

The performer knows where to grip the tube, holding onto the top portion, near the paper rings. This offers the most support. He lifts his feet off the ground slowly. Once he shifts his weight onto the tube, he can even make some small movements.

Hammering Nails with One's Palm

A plank with some nails hammered into it was displayed before the audience. The Qigong master held another nail in his right hand. The master made a loud cry, and the audience saw that the nail in his right hand had been driven into the plank. He drove four more nails into the plank in the same manner, and won a thunderous applaus. He then pulled the four nails out with his bare hand.

The audience saw that his hand was wrapped in a handkerchief, but they did not know how simple this was. The plank is a kind of water-soaked light wood, such as poplar. A young, strong man can easily drive a sharp nail into such a plank with his bare hands. It is very clever to avoid dry, hard wood. It is even easier to pull a nail out of the wood. Performers usually do not pull out the nails they have just inserted; they pull out different nails, which have already been loosened.

Ten Diagnoses of Diseases of "Qigong Super Abilities"

Qigong is a kind of breathing exercise. According to traditional Chinese medical theory, the "Qi" in Qigong is not only the air people breathe, but also the vital energy in the body, which is also called "genuine Qi," or "internal Qi." This "vital energy" is thought to be equivalent to the body's immunity to disease, its adaptability to the environment, and healing ability. The exercise of vital energy is emphasized in traditional Chinese medicine.

The use of Qigong by the Chinese for treating disease and building health has a history of several thousand years. Qigong, one of the remarkable scientific and cultural legacies handed down from ancient times, has contributed greatly to the health of the Chinese people for generations.

At present, in some parts of the country, swindlers are very much alive. They pretend to be Qigong masters and capable of curing any diseases. They have fooled a lot of people.

What tricks do they often play? Here we provide ready answers and introduce the ten best-known skills that have been practiced by swindlers for some time and under many circumstances. It is "must" reading for those who are interested in studying Chinese Qigong.

Some people don't believe that Qigong could cure disease. They consider it sheer nonsense. Here I raise one question: Why do so many people ask the Qigong swindlers to help them? Are they all fooled by deceitful tricks?

In my opinion, the curing of disease by Qigong may have the relevant elements that convince patients. Take the case of an elderly man. Perhaps he is diagnosed as having heart disease, for aged men usually have this type of problem. When a middle-aged woman comes to a Qigong healer, she may well be diagnosed as having "inadequate rest, nervousness, and weakness of the spleen," and so forth.

You can try diagnosing patients yourself. You'll find that you are very successful. Nearly 90 percent of your guesses will be correct. According to what I have learned, the per capita incidence of stomach diseases is highest among the Chinese. About 60 to 70 percent of middle-aged people have stomach upsets. Besides stomach disease, you can add one or two common diseases in diagnosing your patient. He or she will hardly think you incapable of dealing with his or her disease.

However, this is mere guesswork and requires little skill. There are nine other tricks used by Qigong swindlers.

Using the telephone to gather information about the patient

Wangwu asked a Qigong swindler to examine his father. The Qigong swindler thought it a profitable thing, and therefore agreed. "Okay, but I'm exhausted today. I'll go another day," he said.

After he saw Wangwu off, he dialed 114 (the Beijing Directory Service) and got the patient's office number. "I'd like to speak to Lao Wang," the crook said.

"He's not in today."

"I'm one of his old friends. How is he? . . . In the hospital! . . . Seriously ill! . . . Paralytic! . . . Oh, thank you very much."

When Wangwu came again the next day, the Qigong crook said confidently, "I practiced Qigong just now, and remotely examined your father carefully. He is in the hospital. He can't move. He is suffering from paralysis. Due to crowds of people in the hospital the interference is very strong. I'll treat his disease with Qigong, but I'm not sure whether the therapeutic effects will be noticeable."

Wangwu hadn't disclosed any of this information before. How could the master know the whole truth? This was really dramatic, and he began to believe in the remote-examination treatment.

Sending disciples to seek useful information

Many people were waiting outside a clinic curiously and anxiously, for only one person was allowed to enter the room at a time. Two women were talking to each other. "What's wrong with you?" the elder one asked.

"I have got a uterine tumor. My doctor advised me to have an operation. And what about you?"

"My son is in America. He wrote in his letters that he has persistent headaches. Can the Qigong master deal with such a case?" the elder woman asked.

A middle-aged man sitting beside them interrupted them, saying, "I don't believe that Qigong can cure disease. I prefer to spend ten yuan to get to the bottom of this matter."

An hour later these three people walked out of the consulting room, each satisfied with the Qigong master's reply. The master's disciple contributed a lot to this by collecting information outside in the lobby.

Adapting oneself to the circumstances

A Qigong crook was waiting for a bus. Not far from him two women were whispering. "You're prettier after your operation," said one to the other.

"But the remaining scar is quite long. I have to wear tight-collared clothes. And on rainy days it itches."

"A heart operation is very different from smaller operations. Your husband should put aside his newspapers and hobbies and do more house-chores."

"He has been attending to his father these days. He's too tired."

The crook followed them both onto the bus, and then followed the woman who had the operation onto the subway. He asked her politely, "Comrade, I'd like to tell you something."

"To me?" Her suspicions were aroused.

The crook produced his ID card and a certificate indicating that he had completed special Qigong training. "I'm a Qigong doctor. I can give you some advice regarding your health."

Upon hearing this, the people nearby crowded around him. The woman changed her attitude and listened to him attentively. The crook shut his mouth for a while, and then spoke slowly but firmly. "Not long ago you had a major operation. A scar remains on your left breast, just under your neckband." He made gestures while speaking, and pointed to the woman's collar.

The woman blushed immediately. Half surprised and half worried, she nodded her head. "How did you know?" she asked.

The others on the subway talked at great length. "Maybe he has the third eye," "magic power," and so forth. The crook smiled, listening to the people's fervent discussion. Seeing this, the woman became anxious. "What on earth do you mean?"

"I meant that you shouldn't get overtired. You should recuperate at home. Your husband is too busy these days taking care of you and his father. You felt sorry for him and started to do housework yourself. However, it's not good for your rehabilitation, under such psychological and physical pressure."

All her secrets were known by the Qigong master. She couldn't explain the enormous shock she experienced. She was completely perplexed.

Taking advantage of the opportunity when the patient is reckless

People who have studied Chinese martial arts know that if an opponent attacks you, you had better dodge his fixed hand, and then throw him, using his own strength. Some patients seek medical information blindly. Before the Qigong master speaks, the patient will tell the whole story. Such people are easily deceived. The Qigong crook could repeat the patient's words in a different order. At the end of the conversation, the crook can comfort the patient a little, as in this case.

"Doctor, please give my husband a careful examination," an old lady said.

Since older people usually eat little, especially when they are ill, the crook guessed, "Well, his appetite seems bad recently."

"Right. He's put off by oily food. He had no appetite after his stomach operation a year ago. Does this matter?" Thus the old lady revealed the patient's medical story.

"Wait, wait. I knew that already," said the crook, wishing that all patients were like this kindhearted grandma. "You'd better dissuade him from drinking too much."

"He drinks alcohol covertly. I got angry at this," she quickly responded.

Inferring from this that her husband was addicted to alcohol, he began to use technical words, talking about the function of the liver and the definition of veins, that the woman had never heard before. The grandmother was very thankful to the doctor, and praised him highly to her neighbors. "The Qigong doctor is really skilled." What a poor muddleheaded woman!

Stealing the beams and pillars and replacing them with rotten timber—perpetrating a fraud

I once watched a young man who said he could offer the service of checking for disease for several elderly people at Xuanwu Park in downtown Beijing. He twisted a few matches with his fingers, as though the matches had a miraculous effect. Suddenly he raised his head and said to an old man who volunteered to be examined, "Something is wrong with the lower part of your body, right?"

The old man shook his head. "No, the lower part of my body is all right. I sometimes feel dizzy, due to high blood pressure."

"But the root cause of your trouble lies in the lower body," the fellow insisted.

An old woman was also diagnosed. She didn't agree with the crook. "Although I'm getting old, I'm still quite strong. . . . My legs always ache, not my back."

"Just the same, the disease in your back has a bad effect on your legs," the fellow argued.

When I came up seeking advice, the fellow stole a glance at me and said, "Something is wrong with the lower part of your body."

"Please give me an exact definition of 'lower part of the body.' "

"You've studied Western medicine?"

"Yes," I admitted.

"But my theory belongs to traditional Chinese medicine," the fellow argued.

"I'm a graduate student from Beijing Traditional Chinese Medicine College. Why haven't I heard of this before?"

"This term is from Qigong. You don't know Qigong very well. Traditional Chinese medical treatment evolved from Qigong."

I pressed forward steadily. "I'm working at the Human Body Science Association, engaged mainly in Qigong research."

"Well water does not intrude into river water. I'll mind my own business, and you mind yours. I happen to know Zhang Zhenhuan of your unit, and called on him. He said that I boasted outrageously. Later he refused to let me enter his home. I wrote to him saying, 'Your threshold is high, but I don't care anyway.' "

The fraud was brought to light. I gave the rascal a disdainful look.

Trying to upset the patient

The Qigong crook stared at the patient and kept silent for quite a long time. To the patient's surprise, the crook asked him, "Haven't you done anything wrong?"

The patient was caught unprepared. "No," he murmered.

The crook waved his hand impatiently and shouted, "You can leave now. Next!"

"But doctor, you have not examined me."

"I already examined you. Unfortunately, you are not going to cooperate. In that case, you won't recover. Perhaps the condition will even

worsen." He went on to emphasize, "In fact, I have the power of suggestion. It never tells a lie. If you tell the truth, bad suggestions will retreat,
and the Qigong practice will not have a harmful effect on your body."

The patient then confessed that he had a love affair with a woman,
which he kept a secret from his wife.

"That's right. The law of nature shows no mercy. I've found the root
of your disease. Take it easy. I'll exercise Qigong for you," he said, trying
to ease the tension.

The patient argued that he had this disease before his misbehavior.

"Why have you not straightened out your ideas? Before you acted,
such wicked ideas came into your mind, so you got ill. But once the thing
took place, your illness became more serious. This is nature's punishment."

His words not only pressured the patient, but also confused his heart.
If the patient refused to admit that he had made any errors, the crook
would vary his tactics.

"It may not be your sin. Perhaps the sin is your grandfather's, father's,
or your brother's. The fraud influenced the state of your mind. For
example, one of your family members must have hurt an animal. Go and
ask your friends and relatives."

The patient was agitated and didn't know what to do. He had to
acknowledge a mistake he once made, such as eating pork, mutton, or beef
at a restaurant. He guessed that may have been a sort of cruelty to animals.
But, after that, can his disease be controlled? Who knows?

Venting anger on the patient or visitor

"Doctor, can you make a diagnosis based on a single photo?" the visitor
asked.

"That all depends on you. If you don't trust me, I'll be incapable of
curing his disease."

"Doctor, I trust you. Otherwise I wouldn't have come."

The Qigong crook looked at the photo, murmuring, "The girl is
nearsighted. She often feels tired. Her legs and back ache. Her heart
doesn't work well."

"Doctor," interrupted the visitor, "except for the nearsightedness, she
does not have these symptoms."

The crook shouted at him, "You've broken my train of thought and disrupted my whole magnetic field."

"I can't give other patients exact checkups either."

The crook pretended to burst into rage. Over the next few days the Qigong swindler often mentioned this incident, saying that his "magnetic field has been disrupted." He described his visitor as a troublemaker and a rascal with extraordinary powers, and said that he has had to exert the whole of his energies to fighting off the effects of the visitor who disturbed. Though the disturbance was suppressed, his vital energy was almost exhausted. So if he happened to guess correctly on a few cases, he would say, "Look, it's reflected in my unusual skills and profound and high merit." But if it was pointed out that he was incorrect, he could explain, "It's a normal phenomenon, for I'm fighting off the bad effects."

Preparing the stage

A Qigong swindler was invited to cure the disease of a famous writer of the Chinese Literature and Art Association. That's wonderful, thought the crook. If I succeed, I will gain more respect and further my reputation.

The crook read the writer's biography, reports, and books. He consulted all the relevant materials concerning the writer and his family. He discovered that the writer had heart disease, spleen and stomach disease, and high blood pressure. He collected more information by telephone and through his apprentice. He even discovered some useful clues on the spot. For example, he noticed several medicine bottles on the writer's bedside, and quickly drew conclusions from them.

After the examination, the writer and his relatives and friends were all convinced by the Qigong master's magical skills.

Exploratory talks between a Qigong crook and patient

The Qigong crook observed his visitor carefully. The visitor was very thin, and the crook thought this likely due to indigestion or inadequate rest, or perhaps a genetic factor. He said, "Take it easy; don't be nervous. Relaxation will do you good."

When a patient is critically ill, he usually turns to any doctor he can find. And, of course, he is worried about himself. He may say something like, "Doctor, I'm afraid I have a lump somehwere. I'm terribly upset. I believe in Qigong. Please help me."

After such a confession, the crook can describe the symptoms of disturbed sleep. "You often dream at night. Sometimes you feel dizzy. Your living habits have also changed a lot. Am I right?"

Considering the words very appropriate, the patient nods his head. In fact, it's easy for physicians to make diagnoses, but they don't attempt to create a mysterious atmosphere. Pay attention to the words the crook mentions: "head," "heart," "habit," "diet." No matter what symptoms the patient may have, the crook can use these words in his diagnosis to prove his correctness. Here are some interesting dialogues.

"Doctor, are there any other problems?"

"No, nothing serious."

"But you haven't said anything about my heart disease," said the patient, expressing pity over the matter.

"Haven't you noticed? If I told you that you'd be utterly disconcerted. For heart conditions are closely linked with psychological and mental factors. If I told you directly, the words would exert great pressure on your mind. I had to imply it in a roundabout way." That sounds fair and reasonable.

"Doctor, I had a tumor in my uterus. You haven't examined it."

"I always touch on gynecological disease last. I mentioned just now that some of your living habits have changed, which implied this type of disease."

"Doctor, please see where the trouble is. The physicians of Union Hospital told me there was a tumor inside my head. But I thought they must be mistaken."

"I agree with the hospital's diagnosis. But the condition isn't so terrible; the lump hasn't affected the function of your brain. Don't worry. Anyway, if you feel dizzy, it's a bad sign."

"A gastric ulcer and duodenal ulcer are two of my major diseases. I have been suffering from these for many years. You haven't mentioned that."

A sly smile appeared on the master's face. "You haven't realized yet. To cure your disease, I stressed the words 'diet' and 'daily life habits.' Got it? Isn't this perfectly clear? As soon as you stepped into the room, I examined you and found there was a hole in your stomach. It is easy to find. I tested your comprehention ability."

Such deceitful trickery is often carried out by crooks who call themselves Qigong masters. They pretend to possess strange power and medical artistry to cure diseases. A lot of people in the country have been cheated by their cunning crafts. However, we have already found an easy way to prove which is true and which is false.

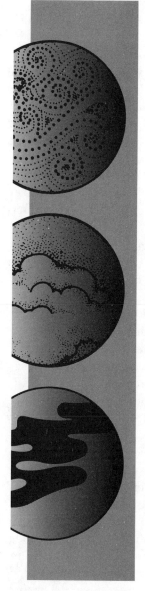

4

The Debate on
Human Extraordinary Ability
vs. Qigong
(Inner Kung Fu)

The Shift in Emphasis

On March 11, 1979, an article appeared in the *Sichuan (Szechuan Province) Daily*, describing "A Child in Dazu County Who Can Identify Chinese Characters Relying on Hearing Alone." This article precipitated a great intellectual debate on "Extraordinary Abilities in Humans," which lasted four years in China. Chinese scientific historians are going to record this dispute as a major pseudoscience event in scientific history.

This debate spread and eventually included all the provinces of China; we can find participants even in remote areas of China, such as Tibet, Xinjiang, Inner Mongolia in the North to Guangxi and Guizhou in the South. The debate originally centered on whether the phenomena of Extraordinary Abilities related to psychic and eventually questioned whether it is related to physics, physiology, psychology, biology, electrical science, statistics, and/or any of about thirty scientific fields.

In all, there were about sixty-eight institutes and thirty-eight universities involved in the debate. According to those scientists promoting the debate, Extraordinary Ability in Humans can involve natural science, mathematics, social science, philosophy, cybernetics, anthroposomatology, and behavioral science.

That the influence of the debate was significant was evidenced by the number of organizations, journals, scientists, and noted public figures that were drawn into the discussion.

It is indeed rare that a psychic phenomenon should generate a debate so intense and which lasted so many years. Indeed, this *is* an event in scientific history.

This debate on Human Special Abilities began in the late 1970s and, after a few years of vigorous debate, receded in importance in academic circles for a few years. This parallels the rise and fall of various investigation and debates on psychic in the West for the past one hundred years. Chinese investigation in psychic is the same; some schools may seem to go out of fashion for a time, but they never disappear.

After several years of theoretical analysis and experimentation, the debate emerged in another form called "External Qigong Phenomena," which was the "second round" in the debate on Human Extraordinary Ability. This new wave of debate and experimentation has some new characteristics. The reemergence of the debate can be traced to June–July 1980, when those who are engaged in the research of Human Extraordinary Ability were preparing the establishment of a "China Anthroposomatology Science Research Society" with the express purpose of publicizing and promoting the research into "Human Extraordinary Ability, Qigong, and Traditional Chinese Medicinal Theory and Their Relationship to Anthroposomatology."

It was pointedly stated that "traditional Chinese Medicine, Qigong, and Human Extraordinary Abilities are essentially the same." The beginning of a surge in interest and media excitement on Human Special Function began in March of 1979. A series of reports on Special Function began to appear, describing people who could use their ear, nose, armpits, feet, or hands to identify Chinese characters (the symbols used to write words in the Chinese language are called "characters") or colors, who could break branches or promote flower growth, locate objects, identify things hidden by blinds or walls, pass through walls to enter buildings, crystal gaze, predict the future, treat disease or do surgery through force of will, cause things to ripen using their minds, and reports of ghostly hauntings, spiritual obsession, gatherings of ghosts, gods or goddesses; appearance of strange pictures in ancient tombs caused scientists to doubt these phenomena and victims and common people to feel unsatisfied at explanations which were given for these reported phenomena. The researchers on special function then instituted a new policy. Under the guidelines of this policy, the Human Science Association (in preparation) was set up; but not admitted by the China Science Association. Then the researchers started their so-called theoretical and applied study stage. During that time, the association called several meetings and proposed that the training and development of special function was the basis of future studies, and classified the special function into two types: (1) the ability to receive and interpret information from the outside environment—such as recognizing characters and colors using one's ear, armpit, foot, hands, and other parts of the body; remote reception of feelings; transfer of thoughts or ideas (mind reading); remote hearing; seeing holographic images using the naked eye; ability to identify in sight-sealed containers; and (2) the ability to change the outside environment—such as promoting flower growth, remote writing, splitting and connecting objects such as match boxes or wire, transportation of objects all by force of mind. In the applied study, the researchers set up a team to study special function and trained a group of "talented individuals (children)" or supermen to explore the human potential which was this Special Function. They regarded a human being as a huge cybernetic system which consisted of many relative stable states. Special function was one of the states. They aimed to study brain function and special function at the same time and find a small number of biological molecular indicators which may be released by the person who has the special function, under different mental conditions, and thus explore the material basis of the special function state. The unification of special function, Qigong, and Traditional Chinese Medicine (TCM) was not only based on the exploration of human potential, but was also part of the group's strategy. In an article entitled "On the Subject of the Scope of Human Science Research" about why there must be a Human Science Association, it stated, "Why are you not a part of the national Traditional Chinese Medical Association; why are you not a part of the Chinese Medical Association, or why are you not a part of a Physiology Association? We have to clarify this point. I thought this over. In the past, the situation was different and Human Science study was used instead of other names. What was human science then? Human science was the study of human special function. Because many people objected to the term 'special function,' and even more misused the term, I changed the term to Human Science. It is more mild and agreeable." In another article by the same author, "Is This the Birth of a New Science Revolution?" the new wording is more clearly explained. "Human special function is unique, perhaps few people can accept it. More accept Qigong because it can treat disease. Special Function cannot amaze a large audience, as Qigong can. Of course, TCM is the most popularized. We can discuss these matters and set up an association to organize and unify the study on Qigong and TCM . . . , so the association can help find new evidence of human special function." More clearly, the author said, "Human special function has been widely studied throughout the world, beginning long ago. We have stepped into the arena later and have poor equipment, but we have a huge advantage. First, we have many Qigongists with dominant special function, other countries do not. Second, we have many descriptions of talents of those who practice Qigong or possess special function in our traditional culture. It is our specialty." These tracts illustrate the necessity of transformation from special function to Qigong.

External Qigong is one special function developed after practice and exercise. This so-called unique Qigong—External Qigong which became popular and spread so widely in China at the end of the 1980s is the second wave of excitement about human special function following the 1970s wave. The researchers on special function, under the pretense of study of TCM and Qigong, told of the strangeness and uniqueness of human special function as they did before. They were of the opinion that External Qigong was released by the Qigongist, and in fact External Qigong was a form of cultivated special function. The high-power Qigongist and Qigongists who have practiced for a long time can identify bodily and underground structures as if using an X-ray, repel attackers and extinguish fire, change biological behavior, can "see" over great distances, cause something to disappear, cut or connect something using their mental force. These are the same things as ESP and PK in human special function. The researchers divided special function into two types: one is spontaneous and often appears in juveniles, the other is what is released by Qigongists who have practiced Qigong for a long time. The Qigongists not only release External Qigong and enter into a sort of "Qigong state," they also can induce others to enter this "Qigong state." That is why the emergence of the popularity of External Qigong was characterized by the appearance of so many Qigongists and Qigong exercise precipitated the onset of special function. When one Qigongist exercises Qigong, he can induce hundreds and hundreds of people to enter a Qigong state (special function state). Among these people, many experienced illusive sensations, illusive sounds, and illusive sights which were regarded as proof of being involved in a "high-power state" (special function state). These Qigongists not only have the above-mentioned powers, they can also treat disease for others and travel in the spiritual world and become a modern medium between the factual and spiritual worlds. To prove the relationship between Qigong's material (physical) basis and the basis for special function, there was a description: "When Qigong enters a high-level stage, the Qi is not limited to inside the body, it can be released from a mind-ordered location or acupuncture point. The Qi is a physical material and contains information. The Qigong at such a high level can be used freely. The External Qigong from different Qigongists is different in quantity (strength) and quality (features). External Qigong can be measured using scientific instruments and shows different effects when examined using instruments with different specifications. Some are ultraviolet rays, some are microwaves, some are electronic particles of measurable power. So I (the author) conclude that the results of the measurements are the derivatives of Qi (External Qigong), not the Qi itself. The Qi can influence matter which is living or dead; for example, another human being. After accepting the Qi, the matter will return information which has a physical material component. The high-power Qigongist can accept the return information in a mind-ordered part of his or her body or acupuncture point; then the information is sent to the brain which analyzes it and forms a sensation.

The application of special function by the young people with special function also is following this process. Finally the sensation appears in the part of the brain which controls sight, so one 'sees' an image as the result. The ability to recognize characters or pictures using the ear, through the skin, 'X-ray vision,' and remote vision all may be involved in that process. In the same way, high-power Qigongists can feel the Qi which is released by other Qigongists and can interpret the shape, color, and feature of the Qi after their brain receives the impulses and analyzes them. As to remote sensation, it is a similar process except for different media." (See "Basic Research in the Development of Human Science," *Nature* 7 [1981].) All of those statements convey the general idea that the physical basis of spontaneous special function and special function induced by a Qigongist are the same; only that one is congenital and the later is developed through practice. That means the Qigong which only helps strengthen the body is not included in the field of special function, and consequently not in the field of Human Science. The researchers on special function and clearly stated: "As to the role of Qigong in health care, body strengthening, that role is not to be included in the field of special function." Clearly the Qigong in which the researchers were interested is only External Qigong which induces special function and is called psychic Qigong by the common people. So the unification of TCM, Qigong, and special function does not mean all aspects and meanings are the same, but is based on the unifying mechanism of special function.

Qigong: The Key to Opening Human Potential

After transforming and broadening their scope from special function to Qigong, the researchers on Human Science began to exert great effort of the study of Qigong. They took Qigong as the key link in the unification of Qigong, TCM, and special function, and as the access to the key feature of Human Science. Qigong is not only related to special function, it is also related to traditional Chinese medicine (traditional Qigong is the source of TCM). Focusing on Qigong is to focus on the practice and theory of Human Science. Exploration of the human potential is the applied Qigong study. The researchers considered human beings to have great potential abilities, which are not explored, like a closed lock. This exploration they called the fourth task of medicine. Qigong is the key to opening the potential. By inference, ancient high-power Qigongists had special function abilities, and ancient pharmacologist and doctors may have been high-power Qigongists. As a derivative of the above idea, the researchers on Qigong can determine types of psychic Qigong which can seemingly facilitate communication between supernatural beings and human beings. They often said, "What are supernatural beings? They are high-power Qigongists. What is a human being? A human being is a huge, complicated system and can be in many relative stable states, such as the waking state, sleeping state, state of stress, hypnotized state, and other special states, such as the Qigong state or special function state. Both the supernatural function or human special function can be induced by practicing Qigong; which can make a human wiser and activate human potential." The researchers concluded that the development of human potential could help to reform China's education system and education methods. China could have eighteen- to twenty-year-old masters. They presented the idea that if China wished to become strong, China would have to progress in the development of human potential which is related to Human Science—special function and Qigong. They also indicated that extraordinary feats Qigongists had done could be done by common people if they continued practicing Qigong. A long time ago, supernatural beings were only in our imagination. If we stress the application of Human Science to cultivate personal potential and find the laws of special function and explore ways to expand this potential, we can say: "Everyone is not only talented, they are also supernatural beings. Some Qigong researchers demonstrated that teaching Qigong in elementary and high schools could make students get higher scores and develop human potential, even create supernatural beings. Furthermore, they presented a hypothesis on Qigong science technique in which they postulated that Qigong Science technique is the most important and advanced of all sciences, which could begin a new revolution in science and technology. One author who wrote a biography for a famous Qigongist, Yan Xin, bragged about special function and Qigong. He described a bright future which would be produced by Qigong and special function from the angle of natural science, philosophy, sociology, psychology study of human intelligence, art, and cosmic science. He wrote: "It is great that special function and Qigong have induced problems and questions in Science. If everyone's potential could be explored and everyone had the ability to transfer thought and the ability to move or remove objects from place to place, then there could be no secrets in anyone's mind because they would know what is in the mind of another and vice versa, and property and law would lose their meaning because everyone could remove things without limitation of time and space. At that time, society would be in chaos, relative to the order, and would produce a new order, morals, and law. Everything in our world is the obstacle of the production of special function. Conversely, special function would destroy everything that exists now." The author further explained the significance of the development of Qigong state, special function state, and special thinking state through practice: "Having the ability to enter those states, we could have what we wished, we could control the cosmos with our minds. If we thought about a Galaxy, we could travel there and influence that place." He even considered Chinese myths about traveling in the air, controlling the winds and falling rain, passing through walls to enter other rooms, telling the past and future, the ability to observe internal body structures like an X-ray, remote hearing, the ability to diagnose disease, methods of opening locks, shrinking one's body, hearing and seeing without the use of ears and eyes, and others as fact. He said, "Now why do we not simply admit the evidence of the reality of those myths? We completely believe that those myths are true." The researchers on Human Science considered that the application of Qigong and Special Function in education and personal cultivation would produce more talented people in the twenty-first century. At that time, China would be on top of the world in Science and Technology. How beautiful a future it was to be!

Qigong Miracles and Special Function

Qigong—the bridge between special function and human science—spread all over China with all its attendant peculiarities at the end of the 1980s.

For clarity's sake, here we only talk about External Qigong or psychic Qigong (the essence and history of Qigong has already been discussed in chapter 1). This type of Qigong was hyped by researchers and became the focus of Human Science. That kind of Qigong was featured as the source of power of some events which illustrated human special function. Here we do not want to compare Qigong with special function on a point-by-point basis when we unveil the truth behind the so-called Qigong miracles. But the following are some real events.

The effect of External Qigong on living and nonliving things (PK phenomenon in special function terminology)

It was reported that External Qigong can make a rabbit's heart beat weaker and weaker, and eventually make the heart stop beating after irregular patterns. In another instance, a Qigongist indicated flowers in bud, and after radiating External Qigong, the flowers burst into bloom. It has been claimed External Qigong can change human heartbeat rate, temperature, and blood pressure; cause instant weight loss; decrease intraocular pressure; and elongate or shorten fingers. Among these, causing flowers to bloom and stopping a rabbit's heartbeat have been proven false (announced in *Qigong and Fraud*, published by China Medical Technology Press), the remainder are the result of suggestion or hoax (announced in *Exposure of Pseudo-Qigong*, San Wan Press).

Remote killing or control (in special function— using the power of the mind to cut or move objects)

A Qigongist declared that he could radiate Qigong while talking, and this Qigong contains biological information which can induce people in the audience to accept this Qigong information and instruction. The audience then exhibits a variety of responses—crying, laughing, dancing, talking, erratic or nervous behavior, some may fall into a coma, etc. One so-called super-Qigongist's lectures attracted thousands of believers. Yan Xin said he taught Qigong to thirty thousand believers. The lecture later turned into an exercise of remote radiation and reception of Qigong. The Qigongist declared he could discharge biological electricity (in the frequency of 10 to 360 MHz, work power, 30 to 65 dBm, an electromagnetic wave with high frequency and low intensity) which can control human behavior.

Remote killing is an example of External Qigong fraud. One female soldier, who said she did not believe in this kind of Qigong and dismissed remote killing as a hoax, was told by a Qigongist: "I will radiate remote Qigong at 9 P.M. today. Please wait in your room." When that time came, the soldier suddenly felt a shortness of breath. Her breathing became irregular and she became dizzy, and then her breathing stopped and her heartbeat stopped. She awakened two minutes later. From then on, she declared, "It is really true!" in a panic, and the Qigongist became famous. He stated that remote killing can treat disease and could either protect people or kill people. This event set the conditions for fraud and caused people to accept this power as real. "Super-Qigongists" emerged through such hoaxes. In fact, remote killing is nothing but a fraud. The soldier was influenced by suggestion from the Qigongist and has a weak psychological tolerance of outside influences. If the Qigongist really had the ability to kill someone from afar, and could radiate such a strong electromagnetic wave (30 to 65 dBm) capable of injuring someone, why did he set a time when this was to be done? If he wished to retaliate against the soldier's disclaimer, he could have done so at any time (exposed in *The Modern Wizard and Magic Woman*, Culture and Art Press).

Removing watch needles, curving keys, moving objects, cutting steel bands, and performing surgical operations using mental power

These kinds of events are commonly reported in parapsychological material from foreign countries. It is a shame that the methods and content of External Qigong which spread throughout China followed the same old practices. Those kinds of tricks have hoodwinked thousands of people.

One Qigongist, who said he could do surgical operations using the power of his mind, set out to demonstrate this. He put a piece of white cloth over the patient in the area in which the operation was to be performed, assumed a serious pose as if to "radiate" Qigong, and was handed a knife to make an incision. The audience saw blood flowing as in a real operation. He then appeared to put his hand inside the patient and took out some material and told the assistants and onlookers to watch carefully. He told them this material was diseased tissue, and now that the diseased tissue had been removed, the patient would recover, and he threw the material away. The Qigongist appeared to radiate Qigong again for a time to repair the incision. When he removed the white cloth, the incision seemed to be completely healed, and one saw only normal tissue without any trace of an operation. During the operation, the patient felt no pain. This is a magic show and should fool no one. The fact is the white cloth is a foil. When the Qigongist picked up the white cloth, he also grasped a pig bladder filled with blood and a small piece of animal organ hidden under the cloth. When he put the cloth on the patient's body, everything was ready and in the correct location. When he pretended to be making the incision in the patient, he cut the bladder and the blood in the bladder began to flow out. What he "removed from the patient" was the small piece of animal tissue. Such Qigong is completely a fraud. Professor Song Tianbin, who exposed this fraud and is working in the Department of Qigong, Beijing Traditional Medical Institute, is often filled with indignation when he speaks of these events. He says this type of event not only defames Qigong; more regrettably, the immoral Qigongist also lost his ethics in the pursuit of wealth, and delays the treatment of patients who need medical attention.

As to curving keys and spoons using the power of the mind, this trick performed by an Israeli-born alleged psychic was exposed by a magician in the 1970s. At first, the Israeli declared it was a phenomenon of special function and he performed this trick all over European countries and America. Such old-fashioned magic was performed in China by some Qigongists. Other tricks such as removing watch hands, shrinking objects, and cutting steel by use of mental power are also really magic tricks— skill and hoax combined.

Mind reading (thought transfer in special function)

Qigongists declare they know what people are thinking. One Qigongist from Beijing gathered several friends together and performed thought transfer and mind reading. After hanging up four pictures which were of a black cat, white rabbit, yellow dog, and red fox respectively, the

Qigongist produced four sealed envelopes which contained the above pictures respectively. He told his friends he could take the pictures out of the envelopes and the pictures would be the same as they had in their minds or he could make them think of one of the pictures as he wished and then he would open the envelopes and compare that picture with the one he ordered them to think about. His friends, after being involved in such tests, were surprised at the completely correct results, and praised the Qigongist's ability—special function. As a matter of fact, the Qigongist had neither ability nor special function, only skill at fraud and general magic. In this performance, there were two required conditions: one is that he ask which picture his friends were thinking about. The other is that he open the envelopes himself. Under the two conditions, the Qigongist could deceive his friends successfully without a mistake. The sealed envelopes had four layers which contained all four thin pictures identical to the hanging pictures. It was difficult to see that there was something different about the envelopes, because the envelopes were thick and the pictures were so thin. When his friends told him which picture they were thinking about, the Qigongist took out that picture immediately by sleight of hand after opening the layer which contained the picture. So he was right time after time. That kind of mind reading is not related to Qigong and special function, only magic, using the magic envelopes (exposed in *Exposure of Pseudo-Qigong*, San Wan Press).

Special visual abilities acquired by practicing Qigong (seeing supernatural vision in special function)

Qigongists declare Qigong can give persons the functions of extraordinary vision, sight, hearing, appetite, and even the ability to see supernatural beings after practicing Qigong for a certain time. If you had those functions, you could see what others could not see, hear what others could not, and talk with supernatural beings. Zhang Xiangyu, a super-Qigongist who gained considerable fame among contemporaries, supposedly can talk with the supernatural world. In *Great Natural Soul*, a biography of Zhang Xiangyu, there are many statements about those extraordinary things. We can give no more detailed examples here because of the limitation of space. This type of magic was spread in European countries and the

United States in the nineteenth century. The soul medium was a Qigongist who had spontaneous (innate) Qigong. The soul medium in this case differed in that his ability was acquired by practice. It is a pity that those Qigongists can associate such fraud with Qigong. The facts inform people to examine the process again. In fact, in Zhang's case, the functions were a complete hoax except she had illusive feelings because of her incorrect method of practice of Qigong. She admitted that point after she had been put in jail with the charge of deceiving people.

Telling the future and reliving the past (fortune-telling in special function)

Some Qigongists boast they could tell the future after practicing Qigong. Those who bragged about this called the ability a superability, because it is free from the limitation of time and space. Super-Qigongists can supposedly enter fourth-dimensional and fifth-dimensional space. In this space, their sight and behavior are not limited. Once Qigongists judge and feel they have overstepped time and space, interval and obstacles become nothing. Given this criteria, one would be led to believe that special function of passing through walls and entering locked rooms is also possible. It is as if the Qigongists have uncovered the other side of the truth and become supernaturals. Their statements are very interesting, but let's expose what they told about the future.

They rely on the art of analyzing dreams, telling about danger, tragedy, disaster, and their deductions from dreams; telling the order of decorated objects; telling the location of a car after it had been driven for twenty minutes; telling the plays in a game of chess—all involve a combination of facts and logic. This type of fortune-telling seems to defame the Qigongists. A super-Qigongist called Zhang Hongbao claims he knew the meaning of the congenital mark on the head of Gobachev. He said the mark was a map of Europe. He explained that the spots surrounding the main mark were the countries of Europe. The darker-colored spots indicated countries that would experience conflict or disaster. Then he gave his interpretation of the European situation. As for Romania, he said the president's reign was over. Hearing this type of fortune-telling, one does not know whether to laugh or cry. The motivation for this type of announcement is either completely far-fetched, foolish thinking, or else purposefully turning a simple thing into a mystery. It is difficult to clarify. This type of simple fortune-telling does not require talent nor Qigong practice. It just requires one to call attention to strange shapes or peculiar phenomenon, and the use of serious, equivocal language. As to who will become a leader or which leaders may step down or who will face disaster, one must have good general knowledge of the world and be familiar with some ancient astrology. There is no connection between telling the future and special function.

Summoning the wind and rain
(special abilities gained by practicing Qigong)

It was an astonishing story that spread all over the world about extinguishing the Daxingan Mountain forest fire. This is the story as told by the Qigongist's eulogists. The Daxingan forest fire was huge, and not many disasters could compare to it. The Chinese government sent equipment, policemen, firefighters, and thousands of people to help extinguish the fire. The wind was helping spread the fire, which got bigger and more intense. Thousands of acres of forest were burning. The firefighters achieved small victories, but the fire fought back and claimed many human lives. Every technical method was used to fight the fire, including artificial rain dropped from airplanes. At the same time, some institutes invited Mr. Yan Xin to help extinguish the fire through radiation of Qigong which could summon wind and rain. To prove the magic function of Yan Xin was real, the following conditions were agreed upon: (1) the time the rain would fall would be indicated by the organization, (2) the weather at the appointed time should be clear with no cloud, (3) that the area of precipitation should be delineated, and (4) the time the rain fell should be the same or close to the time Qigong was given out.

The experiment was begun. Yan Xin radiated Qigong in Beijing, while the fire was burning in Daxingan Mountains, 2,000 kilometers from Beijing.

The east line of the fire was still burning with the help of prevailing winds and was quite intense although it had been extinguished several times.

The leader who was in charge of extinguishing the fire was the division commander of the Shenyang Military Command. The commander had a military phone connected directly to Beijing.

"How is the weather there now?" asked Beijing. The commander said, "Fine. Sun shining, no clouds." Yan sat and talked with people and calmly said: "Tell him rain will be falling in twenty minutes." The information was immediately conveyed to the affected area in the Daxingan Mountains. The commander ordered his men happily, "Keep up observation. Rain will be falling in twenty minutes." Yan was still talking calmly and easily about something related to Qigong and other subjects. He gave out Qigong through his mind, not by action. While he kept talking, Qigong was radiated to the spot.

After ten minutes, an exciting phenomenon occurred in the area. Clouds appeared. It was peculiar. The commanders in Beijing were very happy. However, Yan was still calm and continued to chat with onlookers. "Rain will begin falling in ten minutes. Keep up your careful observation." It was at that time, twenty minutes into the event, that a cold wind began to blow and rain began to fall. The rain became heavier and heavier, and the firefighters and local people responded by cheering and raising their hands.

The rainfall lasted for forty-eight minutes, then stopped. The fire was under control in general, and more than half of the forest fire was extinguished. Only a small section was still burning which was easy to extinguish.

Everyone who heard this story was moved. After thinking it over, though, one realizes this was merely a magic show and would be an interesting story if told as a joke after dinner. How could Yan give out Qigong while calmly talking to onlookers, let alone the huge power needed to accomplish such an event? How could he really summon that rain? The author of the report was so famous, how could he believe such a magic story so easily? It is worth examining the event. Yan himself said extinguishing the fire was a failure because of many factors. Here there is no need to help Yan make an explanation; it is important to think about why he could not have accomplished extinguishing the fire and to tell his believers never to be deceived by this so called exciting news.

Smoke emanating from hands (high-level function in special function)

Some Qigongists declare one can see them radiating Qigong if their Qigong is of a high level and high grade. One Qigongist made some movements, then let the audience watch his fingers. Some exclaimed they saw a red light, some said it was yellow, and some said it was gaslike with white rays. To a professor who has studied Qigong for a long time, such a hoax was a puzzle. After careful observation and study, he finally found the key. There was white phosphorus on the Qigongist's fingernails! Phosphorus is an element with a low ignition point. It easily gives out smoke and light without flame after being rubbed with the palm. That was the magic of the Qigongist. The "burning clothes of Qigong" trick performed by Zhang Baosheng, a super-Qigongist, was accomplished this way.

There are many similar "miracles" reported and spread among the people. There are many books about such magic on bookshelves, such as *Super Qigongist Emerging, Super Qigongists, Great Natural Soul*, and *China Supermen*. There are tens of "miracles" in each book. It seems there are hundreds of "miracles." I am only selecting several from the "sea of miracles."

Four Chinese Contemporary Super-Qigongists: Yan Xin, Zhang Hongbao, Zhang Xiangyu, and Zhang Baosheng

Chinese Qigong has a long history and has been passed down for thousands of years. It is divided into many sects. Basically, it can be divided into hard Qigong (characterized by the seeming ability to cut metal and swallow knives and by fighting) and soft Qigong (used for health care and treatment of disease). From the late 1970s it was replaced or mixed with special function, and the trend became very strong in the middle and late 1980s. Not only were there many sects of Qigong which claimed they had been hidden for a long time, so-called congenital, original, or native Qigongists also emerged to perform. The different levels of national Qigongists and their believers constituted a strong force in Chinese society at the end of the 1980s. It was said by an expert on Qigong study that the types of Qigong increased about three hundred kinds a year. It has been estimated that there are about ten thousand types of Qigong in China. Among them, the most well known are the Qigong practiced by four contemporary super-Qigongists: Yan Xin, Zhang Hongbao, Zhang Xiangyu, and Zhang Baosheng. The fame of their Qigong spread everywhere in

China and other countries and they received high rewards and great fame. These super-Qigongists have thousands and thousand of believers, among them the most powerful people in Chinese society. They had organizations dedicated to them, medical units, and publication houses that published biographies of them: *Great Qigongists* (Yan Xin), *Great Qigongist Emerging* (Zhang Hongbao), *Great Natural Soul* (Zhang Xiangyu), and *Supernatural Baosheng Zhang* (Zhang Baosheng). There are many other books and publications about their "magic" Qigong. Millions of these publications were in circulation after several editions. They counted among their believers top leaders and common people. Their believers may have numbered one hundred million or more. They were considered supermen, and were also millionaires. The following are brief true biographies of them.

Yan Xin, male, was born in Sichuan Province, graduated from Chengdu TCM college in 1977, and then served as a teacher in Mianyang TCM school. He often prescribed strange remedies, such as treating disease by drinking cold water, eating noodles, drinking vegetable oil, and other non-medicine. He became a professional doctor in the out-patient department of Chongqing TCM Institute in 1982. In less than two years, his medical license was revoked due to his odd superstitious practices. Then Yan hunted everywhere for work, and became a quack doctor. It is strange that Yan's name became famous, and within several years he became known as a super-Qigongist, a Qigongist with special function from his beginnings as a quack. His outstanding power is the supposed ability to treat disease from a different location (remote-control treatment). It has been reported that Yan diagnosed and treated patients a thousand times with a 95 percent diagnosis rate, a 65.8 percent dominant effect rate, and a 42 percent instant effect rate. Yan used the following ways to "remotely control" disease treatment.

1. Integration of Qigong therapy and TCM therapy
2. Prediagnosis and treatment of disease by drinking water
3. Diagnosis and treatment of disease by Qigong and correspondence
4. Diagnosis and treatment of disease by telephone
5. Diagnosis and treatment of disease by talking with the patient

In July 1984, the *Sichuan Workers' Daily* newspaper began to report Yan's magic Qigong and published a long article entitled, "Magic, Medicine,

Mystery, Reality." From this, Yan became famous all over China. The reports on "Instant Disappearance of Tumor," "Comminuted Fracture Cured Instantly," "National Defense Technology and Engineering Committee Invites Yan to Treat the Tumor Suffered by the Great Man Who Made Atomic and Hydrogen Bombs," "Yan Lowered the High Temperature and Saved the Patient," "Yan Called the Wind and Rain," "Yan Changed Water Molecular Structure from 2,000 Kilometers Away," "Yan Extinguished the Fire on Daxingan Mountains from 2,000 Kilometers Away," and others spread quickly. In 1986, Yan was called to Beijing and performed his magic Qigong and magic medicine. Within months, top officials, common people, and soldiers all asked Yan for help and wanted to be treated by his Qigong.

At that time, many people from other cities came to Beijing because of Yan's fame and waited for Yan's magic diagnosis and treatment. Yan indeed gave his best and used his strange medical ways which he invented, from giving "Lectures with Qigong" to "Remote Treatment of Disease." These days were very exciting; every report was greeted by fervent listeners. The Qigong Science Association delegation was invited to visit Japan under the lead of Zhang Zhenhuan. He invited Yan along as a special guest. After Yan returned to Beijing, there was an astonishing news report, "Fighting in Tokyo Using Qigong," which said Yan beat a Japanese super-Qigongist and made him drunk by increasing the wine the Japanese drank; Yan changed soft drink, water, and tea in Japan through his Qigong; Yan cured the Japanese man's old elbow injury on the spot. Those reports gave Yan his first superclaim to fame. The second was gained through scientific investigation of his Qigong. From December 1986 to January 1987, the Qigong study group at Hsinghua University conducted an experiment of Yan's Qigong as it effected change in water molecular structure. The result, which was published on behalf of the group, shook the academic field all over the world. Yan then became known as a supernatural, highest-level Qigongist. Even the persons who conducted the experiment became famous. However, the Department of Scientific Administration at Hsinghua University and other doubters expressed skepticism about the scientific validity of the experiment shortly after the result was published. Thus Yan's reputation suffered for the first time. That kind of experiment was actually a pseudoscientific test (the details will be discussed in chapter 5). This was Yan's first defeat.

The second failure of Yan concerned the treatment of the tumor of Deng Jiaxian, who was the founding leader in the production of the atomic and hydrogen bombs. Deng suffered from rectal cancer and underwent an operation in 1985. He suffered a relapse in 1986. Concerned about his serious condition, some suggested inviting Yan who had cured Deng's high temperature during a previous illness. At that time, Yan was not a common Qigongist. He was a super-Qigongist who supposedly had magic abilities. Stories in circulation reported that Yan had cured many kinds of difficult diseases, especially tumors that were cured just after Yan radiated Qigong. After Yan received the invitation, he went to the 301 Hospital on June 27, 1986, for the treatment of Deng's disease. From that time until Deng's death on July 29 of that year, Yan used all his magic Qigong and failed to save the outstanding scientist. The facts grimly tell us that Yan had no special magic way to save human life even though he said he could do just that. Similarly the reports on special cures are false. It is known that Qigongists can do nothing about life and death. Ironically, Yan gave a detailed explanation about the failure. He said it could be attributed to the following reasons:

1. Three hundred one Hospital did not give him an official invitation which greatly affected Yan's mood and interfered with his ability to radiate Qigong.
2. During treatment, he experienced much interference, which made the Qigong weaker.
3. The patient did not cooperate fully with the Qigongist. During the treatment, Yan prescribed Deng eat a pig pancreas. Deng did not follow the prescription, which made Yan feel very dissatisfied. Yan said that is what his Qigong ordered; his Qigong made such a prescription.

Yan's third failure was extinguishing the fire in the Daxingan Mountains, already discussed in this chapter.

Yan Xin enjoyed his short-lived fame as a super-Qigongist. Now he is in the United States. What will he be in the eyes of honest Americans? They will either believe those magic Qigong tricks and worship him blindly or stop to think over what is behind his "power." We hope Americans do not believe in him easily and are not fooled.

Zhang Hongbao, male, born in Harbin City, graduated from the
Department of Economic Administration, Beijing Science and Technology
University, is known for his practice of Qigong. It is strange that such a
college student who once was absent for ninety days, and did not graduate
after four years of study at the university, was able to set up a course of
study called "Chinese Healthcare and Intelligence Enhancement Qigong."
Let us read a statement from his biography, *Great Qigong Emerging*:

> There was a bright rainbow and a Qigongist came into this life to bring
> happiness into the world. There was a bright sky everywhere. . . . People
> cried, a god was coming, a great Qigongist is coming. This news shook
> many people because it occurred so suddenly. Within a year this kind of
> Qigong spread all over the country. . . . We have one name to thank for
> the astonishing events produced in Chinese healthcare and intelligence
> enhancement, and that is Hongbao Zhang.
>
> This is Zhang Hongbao. He can change his thought processes so that
> he resembles a god. He has combined a variety of methods and styles
> recorded in History and Literature including Buddhism, Taoism, Confu-
> cianism, Medicine, Gongfu, Folk Customs and Indian Style of Gongfu,
> and Christianity; edited and rearranged these traditions to produce ten
> principles of his special Qigong system as an integrated belief system.

This statement presents Zhang as a supernatural being from heaven
who had ten magic abilities and ten magic powers. He possessed all magic
recorded in history and mystery. He is a cosmic supernatural being. Of
the four super-Qigongists, Yan Xin was discredited, Zhang Xiangyu was
arrested, Zhang Baosheng was out on bond; only one super-Qigongist,
Zhang Hongbao, was still deceiving people. The author who wrote *Great
Super-Qigongist Emerging* reported that he had six million disciples and one
hundred million believers. More and more accolades were heaped on this
man. However, such terms used to describe him—"talented," "intelli-
gent," "international Qigongist," "peculiar Qigongist," "Super-Qigongist,"
"Strange One," "Qigong manager," "Qigong educator," "Philosopher,"
"Thinker," "Talented Speaker," and others—did not really add to Zhang's
real reputation. Conversely, those terms were proof that he was turning
Qigong into supernatural superstition and a pseudoreligion. He set him-

self up as superior to shamans and witches and religious figures by taking advantage of psychological factors.

Once Zhang became well known, he had a clear aim: to ensure that people thought of him as a Chinese "Qigong god" and become the leader of the Qigong movement. Zhang had the idea, talked about this aim, and took steps to realize his goal.

Zhang Hongbao had a hard time while at the university because he never put much effort into his studies, economic administration, which was required by the institute who sponsored Zhang to go to the university. "He was often absent and no one knew where he was. He always made reasonable excuses for his absence. It seemed he was honest, but once he was asked questions, he could not answer satisfactorily or talked about irrelevant topics. Every teacher said he did not concentrate on his textbooks or schoolwork," said one of Zhang's teachers. During his college years, he began to put his strategy concerning his special Qigong into action. According to this strategy, he could cut short the old way of others and develop a special art. From this point of view, he got much out of his college life. He learned the tendency of people in academics to regard time as precious as gold; that they do not take time out for health care. He got an idea; if he set up a kind of Qigong which is suitable for the intelligentsia, he would be considered the foremost expert on Qigong. Then he practiced some magic tricks and performed them for classmates and teachers. This proved to be very effective. He fooled many people, and attracted a following. He began to brag about himself and perform his special Qigong for a wider circle. He kept expanding his theory and gave a series of lectures and demonstrations at the university. At first, he performed soft Qigong and "body shrinking." He asked others to tie him up with rope, and escaped by radiating Qigong. (Actually this was low-level magic.) Onlookers were astonished; many wanted to become his students. At first he had about seventy to eighty students, but the number soon increased. He then called for a Qigong research association to be set up, which created a surge in interest in Qigong. His dream was being realized step by step. Zhang became general director of the Qigong Research Association which was affiliated with Beijing Science and Technology University. There, he was able to engage in Qigong performance. His Chinese Healthcare and Intelligence-Enhancement Qigong spread from this university to Beijing University, Hsianghua University, the China People's University, and fourteen other schools and eleven institutes including the China Science Academy, the China Social Science Academy, and the China Agriculture Academy which constituted a significant movement among the intelligentsia. He trained people in class after class. In order to promote his Qigong, he conducted performances everywhere in China. He explained, "In order to let Qigong enter the life of academics, persuade them to join the Qigong field, and make Qigong more easily accepted." He invented a Qigong with fast rhythm which is similar to our modern lifestyle because academics place much emphasis on time and cannot take much time to focus on Qigong. His Qigong took only fifteen to eighteen hours to learn. In this Qigong training, students could learn "pitching Qi," "radiating Qigong," "Kicking away disease," "Feeling light," "treating disease," and other magic included in his "ten magic states" and "ten magic changes." Zhang quickly became a familiar figure in academic circles. *China Culture Daily* reported on November 18, 1987, "Compared to Wild Goose Qigong, Crane Qigong, and other Qigong styles which have been shown before, 'Chinese Healthcare and Intelligence-Enhancement Qigong' is most attractive to the intelligentsia in Beijing's Universities and Institutes. Many of them have made an effort to learn and now practice this Qigong." The *People's Daily* (foreign edition) reported on this Qigong in an article entitled "Qigong Popularity Among the Intelligentsia." Another publication contained a long article entitled "Qigong Stirs Up Science City." Clearly, Zhang's first step in his plan was realized. The second step was to become familiar to the entire press circle. First he focused on the *People's Daily*, and succeeded. Then he taught his Qigong through his intensive, simplified classes to the staff and minister of the Broadcast and Television Department in the capital. This shook news departments all over the country. The *People's Daily* formerly avoided publishing reports on Qigong, but on January 8, 1988, suddenly published a news article about "Intensive Qigong classes held by news and culture departments in the capital." After this, many publications and television and broadcast stations feared being late to report about Zhang's Qigong. Foreign TV station correspondents also came to visit him. Thus, he accomplished his second step. His third step was to affect governmental agencies. This step would greatly promote his Qigong, Zhang said. He set up training classes; had free access to examine people in government, diagnosing their diseases; and in time, gathered many believers and supporters including the Minister of Public Security, judges of the Supreme People's Court, and prosecutor. Thereby, Zhang entered high society. (It is known that one lecture by Zhang Hongbao attracted sixty top officials who came in their high-powered cars to the meeting.)

Zhang became most famous. He was "supernaturalized" as a person, his Qigong was "supernaturalized." His believers could not criticize or resist the supernatural. They believed everything they heard about Zhang's magic Qigong, such as the ability to cure 109 kinds of disease, to summon the wind and rain, to lift an airplane, to transport heavy objects, to remotely diagnose and treat disease, to help with weight loss, to decrease patients' temperature, to change the length of his fingers, to produce smoke from his fingers, to toast food held in his hand, to conduct electricity through the fingers, to kill animals by the force of his mind, to induce special function in his disciples, to change traffic lights based on his own progress in traffic, to hide himself in the air, to make a halo appear around his head. A picture which showed a colorful circle of light around his head was produced and circulated by his disciples in order to supernaturalize Zhang's Qigong. In the picture, Zhang is sitting on a lotuslike cement slab and is wearing a set of black clothing. His eyes are almost closed, and three fingers of his right hand are pointing upward. Colored circles surround his head. This picture is easy to make, using certain photographic techniques, but the picture, used as the cover of *Great Qigongist Emerging,* inspired and fooled many. Even believers were willing to pay a good bit of money to buy the book and the picture. Zhang used the money earned in this fraudulent way to set up International Qigong Corporation and International Qigong University. He became so famous that many foreigners began to believe in him. He conducted magic shows, deceiving people who paid money to watch; assailed women with obscenities; and had no morals concerning use of Qigong science. Not everyone in China could be fooled by his Qigong; there were many academics and scientists ready to expose his fraudulent and deceiving ways.

One who is an expert on Qigong studies wrote a book titled *Exposing Pseudo-Qigong* to unveil Zhang's magic. One scientist said indignantly, "I graduated from a university before liberation and am sixty-four years old.

At the time, the superstitious religion named Yiguandao spread every-where, but secretly. Now some spread openly, using the name of Qigong and special function, put a nice label on it. The situation is intolerable." It is known that many victims are filing suit against the super-Qigongist. What is his future? We must wait to know.

Zhang Xiangyu, female, born in Beijing, was an actress. She is the founder of Nature-Centered Qigong, which was invented through Zhang's fraud on the name of "God." It is said that Zhang, during her practice of Qigong, heard someone tell her that this Qigong named "Nature-Centered" was lost for a long time, and it is her mission to spread the Qigong. She wished to conduct her Qigong in order to save mankind. She said, "This Qigong will go into the world because only it can save humankind. Without it, there would be disaster." "We have to propagate the Qigong rapidly, and let it spread in the world without any secret. The year 2000 is coming. . . . There will be fundamental changes in the twenty-first century. What should we do? The only way to protect our-selves is to conduct Qigong and have it become a super-Qigong in order to bring humankind back to nature. This is the best way to save humankind. Otherwise, we face death and disaster. . . . This is not a joke; time will convince you." How dangerous is this situation? She established her Nature-Centered Qigong, and at the very beginning linked the beliefs with other supernatural phenomena. In order to convince people of her supernatural power, she invented a "cosmos language" in which she used some modern terms. The Qigong's goal was to teach one to have super-natural abilities of feelings, hearing, observation, and speech that others do not have. Thus it could cultivate many talents with many special functions. After practicing this Qigong, you could supposedly see gods' and Buddhas' faces, ghosts, evil beings, supernatural beings, and others who exist only in mystery, and hear statements given out by these supernaturals in order to understand exactly what human life is, and what exactly disease is, and what the future will be. You will know what others are thinking, and you can speak a special language which common people cannot understand but which contains information which can change disaster to happiness, cure disease, and protect against all evils. In the book *Great Nature Soul*, a biog-raphy of Zhang, it was reported Zhang could have dinner with a variety of evil beings; identify hidden persons and objects, some far from her location; listen to ancient music which has disappeared already; illuminate blue light from her fingers after putting her hands into a bowl; and make pictures in magic books become alive. She could know what is wrong with a person's body, and had many special powers. All in all, Zhang was superior to other supernaturals and possessed whole intelligence and functions of a super-being. She had four ways to cure disease.

1. *Dispelling evil*: This is the witch's way which has existed since a long time ago. The witch used some disgusting gestures to show she had summoned some supernaturals and then cured the disease. If she failed, she explained the patient was possessed by other evil beings.
2. *Magic language*: This is an old magic trick. Zhang can supposedly discipline her disciples or doubters through magic language.
3. *Producing "natural" things*: Zhang said, "Great Nature is an inherent native source. There is natural blood, natural cells, natural bone, and other natural material. Everything in the body is from nature and can be formed from nature. When we treat disease, we can get what we want from nature." Zhang supposedly produced blood, kidneys, nerves, brain cells, and other things used in treating patients' diseases this way.
4. *Performing surgery through power of the mind*: Zhang said, "Performing operations requires a knife, acupuncture requires needles. One with special function does not need anything when he performs an operation. He can do an operation through the power of his mind." In *Great Natural Soul* there is an example. "One day, a young person whose abdomen was punctured by a steel bar (producing severe injuries to kidneys and intestines) was taken to see Zhang. Zhang collected his blood together and infused blood at the same time by radiating Qigong. She also radiated Qigong to repair every injury like one performs a perfect operation. When Zhang required a needle, she made a gesture and an invisible needle was available; when she did not, the needle flew away slowly."

Zhang deceived people everywhere in China (Qinghai, Guangtong, Hainan, Jiangsu, Hebei, Henan, NeiMengu, Helongjiang, Beijing) by this Qigong. (In fact, this is spiritualism.) Her best use of the Nature-centered

Qigong was to teach this Qigong. Within two to three years, she taught over one hundred thousand people. For her instruction, she received money and fame. She was elevated to the position of "god and supernatural" by claiming she could summon wind and rain, return launched missiles, get American secret documents and return them without detection, extinguish fire, protect people from earthquake and flood, and make snow fall. She earned 410,000 Chinese yuan (the Chinese monetary unit) from March 18 to March 31, 1990, by giving twenty-seven Qigong lectures; 80,000 yuan through one-week teaching in Sining in 1988 and much more in many other places. Perhaps it was the big money which made people angry, for Zhang was arrested in April 1990, charged with deceiving people and spreading superstition. This supernatural "tide" disappeared, and now people are not paying attention to the magic. However, two bloodshedding events are still in people's minds. In October 1989 when Zhang was the most famous Qigongist, one officer was practicing Nature-Centered Qigong. One day, a tragedy occurred. Because this Qigong was mixed up with magic and superstition and mystery, many people were crazy and some exhibited mental diseases in which they could see evil beings and supernaturals and were guided by the Qigong "information." In order to cure people who developed mental disorders through practicing Qigong, an institute specially set up a clinic where more than one hundred patients were admitted over two years. The officer mentioned above was one of them. After he had kept practicing for eighty-one days, he felt there was a force which controlled him and wanted him to write and do other things. He said Qigong information told him he had to "go to his native hometown to have a quiet life." On the eighty-fifth day, he suddenly said, "The criminal who made reactionary remarks in his unit has been detected, because the Qigong information has told him about it," and picked up a stone which he said was the criminal's stool. Later he also treated diseases for others. Many people thought he might be abnormal, but he recovered to normal behavior after that. He spent the eighty-sixth day quietly. At dawn of the eighty-seventh day, he went over to the railroad tracks where he lay down and let himself be cut into pieces by a train. Another event which occurred involved a female officer of the Chinese Academy of Science. She suffered numbness in her arms for over ten years which was never clearly diagnosed. In April of 1988, she invited

Zhang to treat the disease and received Qigong treatment seven times. Each time Zhang treated the disease by singing and dancing which Zhang said was the Qigong. After treatment, Zhang required the patient to keep practicing this Qigong. On June 12, 1988, Zhang treated the officer by radiating Qigong as usual. This was having no effect, and the officer's husband asked Zhang when she would recover. Zhang responded that she gave out the greatest Qigong and that she would have remarkable movement during her practice of Qigong within two days. "Be careful, don't disturb her when she receives the Qigong." The next evening, the thirteenth of June, the officer kept practicing as usual and suddenly fell down. The husband, according to Zhang's instruction, did not disturb her. Time passed and the husband became worried and called Zhang. Zhang said, "I will transmit Qigong over the phone and she will be awake in fifteen minutes." The husband waited. After fifteen minutes, his wife was still lying on the floor. At that time, the husband still did not send his wife to the doctor but called Zhang to come to the house. Zhang came and radiated Qigong as usual, which of course had no effect. After over one hour, she was still not in a hospital and was being treated by Zhang Qigong. The husband finally became convinced this was having no effect and brought his wife to a hospital. The doctor said, after examining the wife, "Why did you bring a dead person here?" Who was responsible for the death? Although Zhang is responsible the most because she should not deceive and abuse people through magic and superstition, what about the husband? Why did he believe Nature-Centered Qigong could save life, even revive a dead person, and did nothing to take care of his wife when she was in a coma, until she lost her life? Where is the responsibility?

Zhang Baosheng, male, graduated from junior high school, and was a worker. He was the most notable of the four super-Qigongists because he attained a high position and high pay. Zhang was considered to have innate special function. He was invited to Beijing in May 1982, at the end of the first dispute on special function. In order to stay in Beijing, he served "top officers." On May 18, 1985, he gave a performance of recognizing characters using his ears to Marshal Ye Jianying. Ye praised him and he received a special passport by which he could go to important places. Ye ordered that Zhang receive excellent pay and living conditions. The praise from Marshal Ye made the news and the researchers on special function spread the word

and bragged about his Qigong. Within a short time, Zhang Baosheng was
well known to the people of Beijing. He was invited to show his abilities—
naked-eye X-ray, treatment of disease, locating lost objects, forecasting the
sex of a fetus, performing tricks, and others. He gave many performances,
and believers of special function considered Zhang to have the strongest
special function abilities. An institute also considered having Zhang teach
his Qigong to military forces. The top leader agreed, and he was officially
admitted to the institute. So Zhang could do anything he wanted. He performed his Qigong for top governmental officials, leaders of the military
forces, remarkable scientists, famous actors and actresses, singers, overseas
Chinese, and foreigners. Rumors about this "superman" could be heard
everywhere. At the end of the 1980s, Qigong became immensely popular.
In this wave of interest, Zhang definitely played an important role. Through
his powers he illuminated the special function stage. Although he did not
deliver lectures with Qigong or teach training classes like the other three
super-Qigongists, his position was higher than theirs. He was called
"superman," "supernatural," "person from the stars," "guest from other
world," "living Buddha," "Chinese god," "natural Qigongist," "living god."
More importantly, he received a higher political position and excellent pay.
He had a luxury car, a luxurious home, and servants, which is the condition of top leaders in China. Although all four super-Qigongists were millionaires, Zhang got money from the Chinese government and received
foreigners' gifts, and gifts from the common people. As to his political condition, his car had a siren so as to go through traffic lights freely, and his
briefcase contained a special passport so as to enter top places freely.

The most remarkable features of Zhang's special function was curing
disease and removing things through the power of his mind. He possessed
strong perspective sight like an X-ray. To his eye, everyone was naked. He
was able to "see" through clothes, then skin and muscle, and then into viscera. He received national fame as a super-Qigongist through his new style
of magic performances. He could make people cry with pain, cure
patients with tumors, connect bone fractures, and eliminate boils. He
could examine human energy and circulatory channels and identify
channel changes, detect drugs, locate lost ships under the sea, remove pills
from sealed bottles. He could cause a policeman's watch to be buried in
the earth and an ashtray disappear into his stomach, curve knives and forks,

make whole a torn name card. He could pass through walls and enter other places invisibly. He could make other people's wallets appear in his own pocket; he could set other people's clothes on fire; he could repair TV sets, radios, and VCRs using his Qigong. All and all, it seemed there was nothing he could not do. However, magic is only magic, and it was bound to be exposed someday. The so-called super-Qigongist had to have some faults. Zhang Baosheng, after attaining the top position, could hardly avoid facing someone who never believed in the supernatural and insisted to know the real power behind the Qigong. Faced with this type of situation, Zhang usually dealt with it by diverting the audience's attention and showing some other magic tricks which were not requested by the audience and said to them, "I am such a magic supernatural being, there is no problem to show you my power." Or, he threatened the challenger by bragging he would make the person's trousers disappear or destroyed his watch which finally made the person back down and no longer doubt him. Finally, as in times past with other magicians, the magic was unveiled and many publications reported the news—the cover of mysticism was taken off and the national superman discredited.

In the world news section of the Taiwan newspaper *United Evening Press*, on October 12, 1991, appeared an article, "National Superman Failed," exposing Zhang Baosheng. The article stated, "Recently, Hong Kong film and television stars went to China to give performances to raise money to aid disaster victims in the East. Zhang Baosheng was invited to demonstrate his special function. The result was criticized by the stars."

Zhang's performance was given in secret. The Qigongist Li Hanchi said, "Zhang performed stupid tricks." Zhang Jianting recalled, "The performance was not special function, it was magic, with clumsy movements." Xu Guanwen said directly, "I cannot understand why the nation protects and nurtures such a low-level magician. He performed magic here, using crude actions."

Zhang's special function was very popular in Beijing for over ten years, not because his special function was special and could not be exposed; it was because he had access to top officials' homes and was protected as a very important person. Because of that, it was very difficult to approach him. The doubters had no chance to express any opinion. The persons they wanted to interview were top leaders, officers, overseas Chinese, and foreigners. Those people often suffered from diseases which were very difficult to treat, and wanted to try Qigong therapy. Performing for these people, exhibiting Qigong in a magic way, Zhang not only received a high position, he received official recognition and a special passport which enabled him to deceive people in an official way and receive expensive gifts. Fortunately, among those people there must be some who have never believed in magic Qigong and may defeat Zhang. We can understand why Zhang tried his best to avoid performing among persons who doubted Qigong or wished to evaluate Qigong in a scientific way.

Yuan Zhidao, an American Chinese, is a well-known person in commercial circles. He wanted to meet Zhang when he visited China in 1990. Yuan heard that Zhang could remove something contained in another object by the power of his mind, cause things to burn by touching them, charge a human body with electricity, fill an empty bottle with water, remove pills from a bottle without opening it, and another wonderful skill, make an ashtray disappear into his abdomen. Yuan doubted these skills and invited Yi Shutian to witness the performance together. Yuan announced he would be willing to be the person to have an ashtray put into his abdomen through Zhang's Qigong. If this actually happened, he would have an operation to remove the ashtray and pay US$100,000. Yuan and Zhang made an agreement that Zhang would perform the ashtray trick in the National Guest House on July 28, 1990. The result? Zhang failed, and Yuan exposed this fact to the press. *China Times*, a newspaper published in Taiwan, published an article entitled, "What Magic Did Zhang Baosheng Perform?" The following are excerpts from the article.

> On July 28, Yuan and his friends had made an appointment and had luncheon in the National Guest House. During the luncheon, Zhang went out and came in several times. First, he took a sealed pill bottle, shook the bottle, and a pill appeared in his hand. Then Zhang radiated electricity and touched each one of the guests with his finger, giving them a shock, so the guests would admire him. Then Zhang took two spoons and rubbed them together. The spoons bent into a zig-zag shape, and he threw them on the table. Yuan picked up the spoons immediately and noted there was no change in the temperature of the spoons. Yuan suspected that Zhang might play some magic tricks to avoid radiating "supernatural Qigong."

After the meal, Yuan said to Zhang, "All right, let me swallow the ashtray," and went to sit next to Zhang. Zhang said he wanted to replace the ashtray with Yuan's watch. Yuan agreed.

Zhang went out and came back in as before. He sat down again with the pill bottle and ordered Yuan to hold the bottle. Yuan looked carefully, and found it was full of water. Zhang then took the bottle of water and then began to bring on the supernatural Qigong. He said, "Look, there is water in the bottle." The audience thought the empty bottle had become full and admired Zhang for his trick. Yuan knew it was a magic trick already.

Following the applause by the onlookers, Zhang asked Yuan, "Do you still want me to make your watch disappear into your stomach?" Yuan said, "Yes, without a doubt." Yuan's friends tried to persuade him to give up the test.

A very strange expression appeared on Zhang's face and he did a magic trick which caused some cloth to burn using his empty hand. He then asked Mr. Yi to hold Yuan's watch in one hand. Zhang seized Mr. Yi's hand forcibly, and quickly Zhang picked out the hands of the watch. When Mr. Yi examined the watch, it was indeed missing its hands. The performance astonished the audience, however, Yuan insisted on ingesting the ashtray.

During the confusion, Zhang's entourage began to go out. After doing a performance of recognizing characters behind a wall, Zhang said he had another appointment and had to go. Then he went out, got in his car, and left.

Yuan met Zhang again in a hotel because Zhang had promised to treat a disease of Yuan's friend. Before beginning treatment, Zhang took a long shower. He came out, began treatment, and removed some pus from a lesion of the patient. It seemed astonishing. After Zhang left, Yuan discovered a new piece of soap had been scratched. He suspected the pus could be a mixture of soap and water. More evidence that made Yuan doubt Zhang's supernatural Qigong could be found . . . such as, the same entourage followed Zhang everywhere, appointed places had tools or props which seemed to have been placed there in advance.

Yuan regarded Zhang as a low-level magician if one were evaluating his magic power. After Yuan went back to Taiwan, he sent a letter to Zhang on August 2, and charged that Zhang had destroyed his watch

without permission and demanded that Zhang should reimburse him a
Rolex watch of the same style; and that furthermore, he should apolo-
gize in writing, otherwise he would expose his magic tricks publicly and
hire lawyers to press charges of illegal behavior. In the letter, Yuan also
warned Zhang to stop practicing magic and never deceive people again.

This exposé has illustrated the true nature of Zhang's ability. To say
that Zhang is a low-level magician, is not a sarcastic remark. In fact, the
tricks of "shaking pills from a bottle," "curving spoons," "smoke from fingers'" "burning clothing by touch," and "rejoining torn cards" were
exposed long ago. Unfortunately, Zhang was in a high position and was
protected, and no one could expose the man. The chapter "Supernatural
Beings" in *Exposing Pseudo-Qigong*, published by San Wan Press, exposes
Zhang's pseudo-Qigong. The super-Qigongist has defrauded people
everywhere; how he can save himself, we are waiting to know.

The newspaper *United Evening* reported on Zhang's magic tricks of
using the name of Qigong in an article called "Exposing the Magic of
Supernaturals." It was stated in the article:

1. The props were not examined carefully.
2. The super-Qigongist had a large entourage.
3. The sequence or contents or the performance were not known in
   advance, so the audience could not prepare any props. The performer brought the props.
4. The place was not suitable for the performance, and the audience
   was not able to get a correct angle to watch the performance.
5. The performer never let the audience get a good angle for observation by using some far-fetched reason or words. No picture-
   taking or videotaping was allowed.
6. The performance was too quick to understand the whole process.
   Only the result could be known.
7. The performer often went out of the performing area during the
   performance, using the excuse of Qigong rejuvenation or body
   regulation.
8. The performer and his entourage bragged about supernatural
   Qigong, while actually performing something irrelevant or
   simple.

9. The props used in the performance were not allowed to be tested, or were destroyed immediately.

10. If some doubters demanded some difficult performance as proof, the performer usually performed something else, or refused to do as requested, saying there was something wrong with his body or Qigong field.

11. The performer often started his Qigong performance by exhaling, patting or striking some object; actions which are used in common magic performances.

12. The performer often used some subjective indexes as proof, such as feelings of heat or numbness.

Zhang's Qigong performances exhibit all of the above characteristics.

Reports on Defrauding by Use of Qigong (Special Function)

Since the end of the 1980s, there have been lots of reports on Qigong, super-Qigong, and superforces in newspapers and journals. It has been estimated by a Taiwan newspaper that there were 200 million persons practicing Qigong and an additional 50 million believers since 1989. This, therefore, was a huge movement which spread all over China. The pretend Qigongists and witches were trying their best to invent "supernatural" Qigong to deceive people to earn money. The great popularity of Qigong was, of course, related to the swindlers' magic tricks, and the endorsement of some authorities, but the press and some writers who were involved in Qigong also had definite responsibility because they reported about Qigong performances without discrimination or proper objectivity, producing a sympathetic response in the readers.

Everything is relative. Qigong can cure disease and help people keep fit, and is welcomed by many people, but the swindlers, with the help of the growing popularity of this method, played their tricks to earn the trust of honest people so as to make money and achieve fame. There have been some exposure of their fraud, although the exposures are not as common as the propaganda about Qigong and magic. Here are some reports taken from the *Yuanming World Paper* edited by the Shaanxi Qigong Research Association on October 22, 1991.

On the morning of July 26, 1991, several twenty-year-old Qigongists from Inner Mongolia arrived in the area. They said they could cure any disease and anyone could test their powers free of charge. They soon attracted a crowd. One person came forward saying he suffered from backache and wanted to try Qigong because he had seen no effect from hospital treatment. The Qigongist wearing black clothes spoke some words and moved quickly, then asked for a cigarette-pack wrapper from a bystander, and stuck the paper on the waist of the patient. Then he radiated Qigong through the paper. In an instant, the patient felt heat and pain, and when the Qigongist took away the paper, there was a blister on the man's back. He asked the patient about the pain. The patient said the blister now was painful, but the backache was relieved. The surrounding crowd exclaimed how wonderful this Qigong was. Many with stomach problems, backache, and headache came forward and asked the Qigongists to cure their ailments. Soon, many had blisters on the neck, head, back, waist, and abdomen. One woman who wanted to try the treatment was told by the Qigongists that she suffered from three different diseases, and that they would have to go to the woman's home to give the treatment. After arriving at the home, the Qigongists said, "You must pay us 430 yuan." The woman said, "You promised this would not cost money." The Qigongists answered, "We do not take money if treating minor disease." The woman reluctantly paid the money so she could receive treatment. Another male worker invited them to his home to treat his disease, and welcomed them with cigarettes and good food. However, the Qigongists still asked him to pay 340 yuan, and said, "You have a fast-developing disease. If you do not get treatment, you will die within two months." This statement frightened his mother, who answered with the cry, "We will pay the money, even more."

Du Xiaoshan felt pain from the blister which he received from the Qigongists, and doubted it was the effect of Qigong. He went and followed the Qigongists and watched them carefully. He saw the Qigongists rub some liquid on the paper before they put the paper on the lesion area. Mr. Du determined to try their test again. After the Qigongists put the paper on his skin, Du avoided the Qigongists on purpose. He clearly understood the blister was not caused by Qigong, it was caused by the liquid—a chemical.

Du reported his findings to the local security department immediately, and the department took action quickly and arrested the Qigongists. The facts came out that they had been to Xi'an, Ya'an, Ankang, Yinchuan, and Baotou to make money by cheating people through their pseudo-Qigong. In half a day they had made over 1,200 yuan.

China Sports Paper presented two records of the performance at the "Second International Qigong Conference" which was held in Xi'an in September 1991.

At 2:00 P.M., the performance in the closing ceremony was in progress. Qigongist Song Jiping from Shanxi had sent in a *Qigong Bulletin* which reported a miracle. "Since July 13, Qigongist Jiping Song has done a scientific experiment on Qigong. He can change the congenital code of mosquitoes. In forty-four days, it was estimated that 90 percent of mosquitoes had been changed successfully. He invited people to observe the change in the incidence of mosquitoes biting humans, and that the mosquitoes had begun biting trees, grass, and other insects." Also, it was reported, "Qigongist Song Jiping has shown the highest-level of Buddha nature. he can remotely give out and receive information, and can conquer anything, including himself. If this is true, the world would be wonderful. As to the reality, please discover the answer yourself through your experience."

During the conference, ten Qigongists delivered lectures with Qigong. The audience exhibited strange behavior such as crying or laughing, but no good effects of treatment for any ailment. One paralyzed patient on a stretcher was taken from one meeting to another but all the Qigongists who delivered the lecture with Qigong could do nothing to make him stand up.

A Qigongist from Shanxi confessed to journalists, "At the end of a class on Qigong, people invited me to deliver a lecture with Qigong. I never do this, but because so many people kept waiting, I had to go onto the stage. I talked about the mechanics of Qigong first, and then told a lie. I said that I had phoned a super-Qigongist, and that he and I will give out Qigong together. Then I induced the audience to enter a calm Qigong state. The result was wonderful." After the performance, the Qigongist told the truth. He hadn't phoned any Qigongist. What a lie.

One Qigongist who didn't want to have his name revealed said, "Now many Qigongists cheat people to make money. Mr. Yu created 'Calligraphy Qigong' and made five yuan by writing one character. Mr. Yang bragged he could tell the future and change one's fate by changing your name." One Malaysian, Mr. Chen Yusen, said, "One Qigongist came to Malaysia and asked for 2,000 yuan from students in his Qigong class, promising his Qigong could cure many diseases. But, after ten days, no one was cured by the Qigong."

The book *Qigong and Pseudo-Qigong,* published by Beijing Press, exposed the following cases.

A clinic held by a being from outer space: Chang Wenxia, a then thirty-four-year-old lady living in Natanzi village, Faku county, Liaoning Province, called herself a supernatural lady, goddess, and other names of supernatural beings illustrated in ancient magic books. She said she met beings from other stars who urged her to treat patients and that she would be the medium. So many people from the whole country came here to ask her to cure their diseases. She treated the patients without any inquiry or medicine. She asked the patients to stand near the wall, and gave each a name of a so-called outer-space star-being respectively. The business hours were 11:00 to 12:00 A.M. and 8:00 to 9:00 P.M. During the treatment, the patient would lie on a bed leaving a place so the outer-space being could lie with the patient to cure the disease. Chang made a lot of money cheating people this way. The patients' diseases were not cured or changed, but the Qigong charge amounted to one hundred thousand within two years.

Superforce circle: A priest on the Jiugong Mountain, Hubei Province, said he could enclose a person by drawing a circle with his fingers, even enclose a person who was 1.5 kilometers away, for two hours. Using this superforce circle, he could hasten parturition and make paraplegic people stand up in an instant. One scholar, who was engaged in Qigong study, wanted to experience the superforce Qigong and was willing to be tested by the Qigong. The result showed no effect.

Remote-control treatment: The founder of China Huilian super-Qigong bragged his Qigong was the highest power of Buddha. He could cure disease without touching the patient. If the patient wanted to get the treatment, he need just send in a picture with his address, name, sex, age, and detailed course of the disease. The super-Qigongist could then cure the disease by remote radiation of Qigong. Those who wanted to get treatment paid eighteen yuan, and the Qigongist sent out a treatment card. Patients were advised to exercise according to the information on the card, and received the Qigongist's instructions. So easy it was to make money by claiming to cure disease or help people keep fit!

Information treatment: A Qigongist gave out Qigong to stone, water, prescriptions, and handwriting, and then this material contained the Qigong information. One could take them home and the information could cure disease. The Qigongist charged a lot of money for the material which contained the Qigong information.

Eastern Renaissance

We have a clear picture of Qigong and Special Function in Human Science. The Qigong in Human Science is not the Qigong of traditional Chinese culture, it is the "supernaturalized" Qigong of special function. Qigong and special function are always mentioned together. The transfer from Qigong to special function clearly tells us that special function study has been widened to include Qigong. In 1981, Qian Xuesen predicted that, "Scientific study on human special function will open the lock which binds the mystery of life," and "The practice of special function is leading in this direction (to open the lock). Many new discoveries on special function clearly show that a great revolution in science is coming." Because of the failure of special function study and bad reputation throughout the world, researchers included Qigong study into special function study, and mixed it with Traditional Chinese Medicine, making TCM, Qigong, and special function a unity, so as to pretend to do scientific study and approach these subjects reasonably and be elevated to a higher position in the scientific community. True, special function study, using the name of Qigong study, enjoyed several waves of popularity. The four super-Qigongists emerged during these times; many "supernaturals" with different names appeared. Qigong became thought of as the key of science. From this point of view, special function in the West evolved directly, with spiritism

and life resurrection, whereas the special function in China has its host—
Qigong. Taking advantage of Qigong's role in health care and prolonging
life, the researchers on special function extended its intention and role
without limits.

In practice they put special function ahead of religion. In theory, they
put it ahead of science. In the papers and lectures of Qian Xuesen focused
on special function and human science during the last ten years, he spoke
many times about an Eastern renaissance which will be brought about
through TCM, Qigong, and Special Function in Human Science; and said
this renaissance is the second renaissance, a new scientific revolution, a
greater revolution than that caused by Einstein's announcement of the
theory of relativity. In the "To Establish Set-Up Spirit-Qigongology"
written by Qian, he appraised the good future of Qigong study in China.
He wrote, "In the twenty-first century, an intellectual challenge exists in
the world. If Qigong can promote intelligence, how wonderful it is. Also,
there is proof that Qigong can transfer to special function if one keeps
practicing Qigong. Looking at it as a whole, Qigong can promote the
level of health, and can also promote intelligence. We have enough evidence to prove this. Special Function is related to Qigong. Qigong can
activate human potential. If we promote Qigong study, and make Qigong
scientific, Qigong could enhance our abilities, and our efficiency in
changing ourselves. This is profound research that we should try our best
to accomplish. We should begin by accumulating information and expose
the spiritual Qigong. Then Qigong can become real science. In doing so,
we, the posterity of the Yellow Emperor, should feel no guilt toward our
ancestors. We may attain fame, but for the right reasons." On this immi-
nent renaissance, Qian said, "The twenty-first century will be the time of
intellectual competition. China should work for the future. I think we
will be the model for the world. It will be the victory of socialism.
Because we have adopted Marxist philosophy, it will be a great thing. I
spoke of this at the Human Science Association inaugural meeting
presided over by Zhang Zhenhuan. We must follow this way. It is the
second renaissance. The first renaissance occurred in the fifteenth century,
and it has been five hundred years. We cannot keep following the old
system, we have to create a new system; that is why we call this the second
renaissance." Qian called for members of the Human Science Association

to work together and help each other to cause a new science revolution—an Eastern renaissance. He said, "We recognize our aim—a second renaissance. In the future, we can turn humans into supernaturals. This will be a great advance in human history." Qian thought the breakthrough in human science study should be based on TCM modernization. He said in "The Strategies of TCM Modernization": "Admit TCM (including Qigong, special function) to the modern scientific system, and set up a new human science. Once it is set up, it would promote and reform the present scientific system. It will completely reform this system. We should not only observe phenomena, we should know the cause of the phenomena. This is real TCM modernization. No, not only modernization, adapting TCM for the future. It is a great task. It not only means we will change an old scientific system but set up a new system. It would be a scientific revolution." He postulated in "Special Function and the New Scientific Field": "Qigong theory is connected to TCM theory. I regard Qigong, Special Function, and TCM as a unity."

Researchers on human science hope to achieve a breakthrough in special function study through a breakthrough in TCM study and Qigong study. Qian regarded that when speaking of Qigong, TCM, and special function, Qigong was the most significant. That is to say, in practice, Qigong is the medium of special function. Qigong-Special Function is a peculiarly Chinese invention, and different from special function in the West. The breakthrough in Qigong study (together with TCM modernization) should help to explain the mechanism of special function. It is different from the superpsychologists' work which focuses on relativity and quantum mechanics which eventually comes to a dead end. Chinese researchers on human science are trying a new approach which is the study of the theory and application of human special function. We can say that TCM modernization can aid the theoretical study of Qigong, and Qigong technique can help find real application for special function. Similarly, the breakthrough in Qigong application and success of special function provides theoretical basis for Qigong technique. This is the situation and intent of today's special function study. Qian said in a paper entitled "Unite to Mobilize for a New Science Revolution": "To study how humans mentally interpret the objective world including our own selves, is a very difficult task. To proceed in this study, we have to explore the topic in a new way. I believe Qigong, TCM (including Chinese medicine, Mongolian medicine, Tibetan medicine), and human special function, once integrated with modern science and technology, would create a Marxist Science. This would be a new science. Through this integration, this new science would also change modern science and promote it. This is our great task. Because we would intergrate TCM, Qigong, and special function with Marxism and modern science, it would not be like modern science today. It will be an advancement, a new science revolution. We can say it will be the scientific revolution of the East."

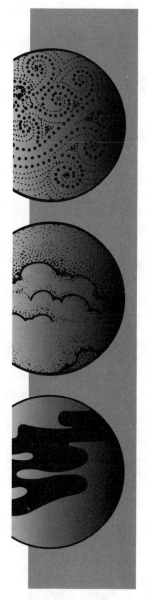

5

Qigong and Ultra-deviation

Ultra-deviation and Its Symptoms

What is ultra-deviation?

Ultra-deviation indicates the psychiatric disorder caused by improper training in Qigong. Qigong is a treasure of the Chinese civilization which can bring benefit to mankind. However, it is neither superhuman strength nor omnipotence. It is a way of preserving health. With appropriate training, it will be effective not only for preventing and treating some chronic diseases and relieving remarkably some intractable diseases against which medicinal therapy brings no relief, but also for strengthening the body and stimulating its potential as well as extending one's life span. Nevertheless, some have become addicted to it, or accept feudal and superstitious points of view. Those overzealously seeking the appearance of "special function" and miracles

137

may be misled and may develop mental disorders. In Chinese, we commonly refer to this problem as "Zou huo Ru mo."

"Zou huo"—going far from the original—is a phrase used by our ancestors to imply that the intensity of the fire and time in the crucible exceeded normal limits when making pills of immortality. The duration and degree is out of control. In Qigong this means the improper level of attainment is reached if the trainee concentrates too intently combined with deep breathing during Qigong training. The symptoms are physical discomfort, unrest, and involuntary movement of the body.

"Ru mo"—becoming spellbound, bewitched—is characterized by anxiety, skepticism, and obsession, which causes the development of improper psychological activities and hence leads to psychiatric disorders. One may accept hallucinations experienced during practice as reality. This may lead to mental confusion or even mania.

According to medical science, ultra-deviation in Qigong is the deviation related to Qigong training. This can be divided into three categories: The first presents itself as purely physical symptoms; the second, psychosis with physical symptoms; and the third, psychosis only. The second and third are more frequently seen with the third the majority of cases. The psychiatric symptoms indicate disturbance in sensation, thinking, emotion, and behavior which occur as a result of the improper practice of Qigong. Improper practice of Qigong includes selection of inappropriate types of Qigong, improper approach to practice, exceeding a reasonable time limit, poor psychological state, and physical and mental diathesis (including whether one has a history of mental disease, a family history of mental disorders or personality defects). "Ultra-deviation" is an uncomfortable and frightening matter, but one should not panic. One may recuperate as long as it is treated in time. It is best to take precautions so as not to develop problems later.

Symptoms of ultra-deviation

Psychiatric symptoms caused by ultra-deviation when practicing Qigong are rather complicated and can be divided into six categories.

1. Most patients have a sense of energy.

Most of the patients we meet who are suffering from deviation of Qigong say that they have a "sense of energy" (Qi), a sense of the presence of increased energy. This is an abnormal sensation from a psychiatric point of view. This sense can be felt when practicing Qigong to certain degrees. It is considered a sensory disturbance if such feelings still persist after people have stopped practicing. One patient complains he senses an electrical-type charge over his head, which presses down as if a cap is covering his head. Other patients complain of physical discomfort which may be all over their bodies or concentrated in a certain part of their chest, the Dantian region (lower abdomen), or private parts, which cannot be dispelled; some feel their head or the whole body were on pins and needles, experiencing small electric shocks or unbearable paralysis. This is a disorder of sensation because these people do not experience or describe these sensations like normal people. The "sense of energy" cannot exist within the body. It is an erroneous experience of the patient. However, the patients think just the opposite; e.g., one woman thought the Qigong master had taken away her energy and she felt weak, exhausted, and unable to move and hence lay in bed for more than half a year. Another patient came from Mongolia. He felt stagnation in the Dantian region, after he practiced Arhat lying Qigong, as if there were hands and a spherical air mass caught in the area and this remained undispersed day and night. As a result, he felt anxious, thought this was incurable, and wished to die. It must be noted that the description of this "sensation of energy" made by patients is consistent with the Qigong masters' instruction and the "External Energy" and "Internal Energy" adopted by dubious Qigong books.

2. Most patients have hallucinations.

Hallucinations are a kind of unreal perceptual experience. Though the visions seen or heard in the hallucination do not exist in reality, patients think they exist from their subjective point of view. They can see someone or something or hear certain sounds out of a void or receive so-called messages. The psychiatric disorder of auditory hallucination caused by deviation of Qigong is related to the Qigong master's suggestion. Generally speaking, it is easy to distinguish hallucinations with a strong folk superstition content such as one can speak in "cosmic language"; sing "cosmos songs"; talk with Bodhisattvas; chat with trees, insects, and snakes; see

celestial beings coming to earth; and meet dead relatives. It is more difficult to deal with those who claim they have "special function." They can
supposedly penetrate another's vital organs; they can "diagnose" and
"cure" disease. Patients of the latter type don't appear much different from
normal people in other aspects of daily life. The only difference is considered a "special function" which normal people do not possess. So they
experience a great sense of pleasure during the preliminary stage of possessing "potency" and they will be most diligent in practicing and radiating
Qigong to "cure disease." Neither they nor their relatives, friends, and colleagues consider theirs to be an abnormal state. This situation results in
compounding and prolonging their disease.

3. More than half of the patients have delusions.

A delusion is a pathological process and is the result of a disturbance in
one's way of thinking. Though inconsistent with reality, the patients
believe their viewpoints are correct, and they can neither be persuaded nor
corrected. The most common sort of delusion among the patients suffering from mental disease caused by deviation of Qigong is that they are
being controlled. One says, "There is a kind of invisible power which
makes me stroll around this tree." Another says, "Nature-centered Qigong
controls my eating habits and elimination." The patients feel they are being
controlled by some sort of invisible power of involuntary sensation. The
delusion of persecution is also often seen among the patients; e.g., they
believe others will do harm to him and intend to steal his "energy." Others
have preposterous grandiose delusions; e.g., one thinks he is omnipotent,
another thinks he possesses superpowers and can dominate the world or is
convinced of his special mission to save mankind.

4. Most patients are highly emotional.

Emotion is a kind of psychological process; an attitude and corresponding
extrinsic expression which occurs when people perceive a situation to be
a certain way. Joy, anger, anxiety, sorrow, melancholy, fear, and brooding
are the seven main emotions of mankind. Deviant strong emotional
response refers to a sort of pathological expression which exceeds the
emotional range of normal people. Among patients with psychiatric dis-

orders caused by deviation of Qigong, some feel upset and anxious because of the extraordinary "sense of energy." Some feel frightened because of the terror of auditory hallucination. Some feel self-satisfied that they possess "special visual ability," "special audio ability," misled by the experience of their hallucinations. One patient felt astonished and trembled with fear after he heard a voice saying something like "Zhang Xiangyu says your magnetic field is intense and it is a hazard to the city of Beijing" and "The earth will explode in 1997." He eventually lay on the ground and could not stand up.

5. Many patients exhibit eccentric behavior.

Eccentric behavior means that deviant from normal behavior which cannot be comprehended by normal people. A number of patients with psychiatric disorder caused by deviation of Qigong have strange behavior. One patient suffering from problems associated with her practicing "nature-centered Qigong" said her dead mother was coming and would ask her for paper money. Since she could not collect it on time, she was worried and knelt on the ground. Once she took a kitchen knife and threw it at her family members while she was singing and jumping and let them kowtow for her. Though they were able to take the knife away, her husband's arms and hands and her children's hands were wounded by her bites. Another time, she heard a voice telling her, "You can fly," so she opened up the window of the building to jump out. Fortunately, she was caught. We see various eccentric behaviors among these patients. Some climb onto subway tracks, some hang themselves, some bite and scratch people with their fingernails and teeth, some hurt or kill people using lethal weapons, some take off their clothes and lie on the ground to "get in contact with the energy of the earth," some even hear transmitted messages such as which pieces to eat while dining on noodles and cucumbers.

The patients who suffer from psychiatric disorders caused by deviation of Qigong and their eccentric behavior are usually plagued by hallucinations and confusion. After recuperation, some patients recall that they heard a voice which told them what to do, or even forced them to do its bidding. This kind of verbal auditory hallucination is called *imperative auditory hallucination*. The patients with such symptoms are rather dangerous. If precautions are not taken, tragedy may occur.

6. Some patients suffer from obstruction of consciousness.

Consciousness indicates a person's ability to recognize self and environment and the degree of distinction of the recognition. The patients suffering from disturbance in this function cannot distinguish the environment or even themselves. That which fails to make clear distinction of the environment is called *environmental conscious disturbance*. Its symptoms are: consciousness in a somnolent state, the range of consciousness contracts, having difficulty with perceptual judgment toward the environment; hallucinations, illusion, and delusions occur intermittently and are sometimes accompanied by attacks or violent behavior toward others. They may partially or completely forget what happened after consciousness recovers; e.g., an interpreter with deviation of Qigong declared that he is a god of energy. He became talkative and agitated and started making eccentric gestures as if he were catching a snake. In another violent incident, he slapped his wife in the face. Later, he could recall nothing about these two events.

Those who cannot distinguish self are said to suffer from disorder of self-consciousness or possession. These patients declare they have been possessed by ghosts, a god, fox spirits, yellow weasels (figures in folktales), or Qigong masters and speak for them simultaneously in their identity, style, and voice. What they said is closely related to Qigong, e.g., they experience possession by 'nature-centered Qigong' or by Qigong masters such as Zhang Xiangyu. Those possessing them speak through their voice.

Where does the symptom "Sense of Energy" come from?

The "Sense of Energy" is the most common symptom among patients with deviation and it is also experienced by Qigong-practicing people without deviation. Where does the "sense of energy" originate and what is its main character? Disregarding explanations offered by the superstitious, there are two opinions based on scientific explanations.

(1) Based on the study of "Human Science," a human body is a large biological field which constantly exchanges energy with the environment during its life span. Based on physical science, "intrinsic energy" (also called Inner Qi) and "extrinsic energy" (also called External Qi) are synthetic waves generated by the body consisting of sound, light, electric, magnetic, heat, and other particles. These waves may encounter obstacles which

causes wave pressure during its propagation within the body; when it encounters nerve endings, people will experience a kind of sensation; when it is transmitted to the cerebral cortex, it is the "sense of energy."The human body is in a special state while in the process of practicing Qigong. Well-trained Qigong practitioners may, to a certain degree, control and channel these waves, and this can be felt. Indeed, the energy exists and penetration of "sense." People holding this point of view have conducted scientific tests using modern technology. However, their principal goal is to prove the effect of "External Qi." According to comments made by some experts, these tests still lack strict test design, with some factors of a priorism and without duplication. So far as the existence of "intrinsic energy" is concerned, it is only a theory. Therefore, the existence of "extrinsic energy" and "intrinsic energy" have not been commonly acknowledged.

(2) An attempt to explain this phenomena on the basis of physics, psychology, and physiology. The explanation can be divided into three parts.

First, some functions of Qigong are general physical phenomenon, e.g., some Qigong masters may begin a session by saying, "Close your eyes slightly, raise your arms to the same height and distance separating your shoulders in a relaxed state. I will conduct energy to you, and your hands will feel numb." You will actually feel numb after you have followed the Qigong master's instructions. Why? It is not difficult to explain. That is because the sense of numbness has something to do with the flow of blood through the blood vessels. One's arms are normally in a drooping state except when they are in motion and working conditions. Blood fills the vessels in the palms and fingers because of the pressure difference caused by the contraction and dilatation of the heart and the weight of the blood in the arm vessels. Since the normal posture of the arms is hanging at one's sides, one does not have exceptional feeling. When the arms are elevated, there is the height difference from the drooping state. In the hydromechanical sense, at this time it is easy for the blood to flow into the heart since some potential energy in the vein vessel increases, but it will be difficult for blood to flow into the hands and fingers since arterial vessels have lost some pressure, and the vessel walls will have shriveled somewhat which adds resistance to blood flow. In fighting to overcome this resistance, there will be further pressure decrease and that means the blood supply is decreased further. At this time, the hands and fingertips especially, which are the farthest from the heart, will feel numb. (Of course, this horizontal lifting is not under working conditions. In that case, blood circulation is in another state.) Second, psychological suggestion may produce the sensation of "energy." "Sense of energy," certainly, is not as simple as we have described; in most cases, it includes a feeling of numbness and bloating, and even a feeling of the presence of energy itself. This is not a reflection of physical phenomena but of psychological suggestion. Suggestion is a special psychological phenomenon which man possesses and it can have great influence if there is no opposing attitude. One famous and typical test has been conducted abroad using a criminal who had been sentenced to death. The executioner announced that punishment would not be conducted by firing squad, hanging, or electrocution but by cutting his artery and letting the blood flow out until he died. The executioner blinded the criminal's eyes and "cut" his wrist artery. The criminal could hear the drop of blood and for a while he could really be considered dead. In fact, the drops of blood were simulated by that of water, and the cut was made by the back of a knife without any incision. This example demonstrated the strong effect of suggestion.

There is a saying about the gain and loss of energy. Those gaining energy quickly are those people with an earnest and sincere attitude as well as a strong susceptibility to suggestion. The Qigong master teaches or treats patients using language, expression, movements, behavior, sight, and other suggestive approaches. The people with a strong sense of suggestion will behave exactly as the master has suggested. If the Qigong master says, "Put your hands in a position as if you were holding a sphere and I will add to your energy. As a result, you will feel there is a pulse of energy between your hands like a magnet. You can neither draw them back nor join them," it is likely the trainee may feel the virtual presence of energy. The Qigong master then adds, "Please be attentive and sense if there is energy running through your body. This energy will attack the point of infection and cause pain and aching wherever your disease is present." Sensitive people will have this sort of feeling in respective places. (Even those who never practice Qigong may feel discomfort and release of disease at some location, owing to psychological effect.) Third, psychological processes may cause some physiological changes and that is not because "energy" exists. The result of long-term psychological study shows: after receiving suggestions, an individual may not only change the movement of skeletal muscles controlled by the voluntary nervous system, but this may also affect the functions of involuntary muscles (viscera, blood vessels, endocrine glands, etc.) controlled by the involuntary nervous system (also called the automatic nervous system). Many types of Qigong require mental focus on certain parts of the body; e.g., mentally focus on the Dantian region. The trainee's attention is highly concentrated on this part of the body for a long time, and this may actually cause some physiological changes including a sense of pain or comfort and rise of temperature through the constant stimulation of psychological signals. However, it is merely that psychological function causes these physiological changes and this has nothing to do with "energy."

In conclusion, "sense of energy" is not that energy actually enters the body but this is an abnormal perception of sensation. If the sense of energy is too strong and causes anxiety, that is deviation of Qigong. Of course, what we have explained is by no means to deny the positive significance of practicing Qigong. The application of suggestion in medical science is a good psychological therapy. Chinese Qigong has its unique characteristics and it undoubtedly should be further developed and analyzed. Those holding scientific attitudes should be encouraged; whereas those proclaiming superstitious attitudes should be opposed.

Not special function but hallucination

It is well known that there are two different points of view concerning the occurrence of "instinctive potency" (also known as "special function") when practicing Qigong.

"Specific function" here refers to "penetrating vision," "remote vision," "remote control," "thought transference," etc. This also indicates "special visual ability," "special audio ability," "ability to recognize fingerprints," and "conduction of messages." The cause of this state is the result of deviation of Qigong, a psychological process, and is regarded as a kind of psychosis in the field of medical science. This view has been acknowledged by the majority of specialists in the field of Qigong. However, some Qigong masters hold the opposite point of view. They deny that this is psychopathy and maintain that this is "instinctive potency" (special function) and trainees may partially or completely possess the above-mentioned abilities after they have practiced to a certain degree, which is called the "advanced state of Qigong." The hearsay concerning "specific function" has become well known; e.g., certain Qigong masters have remarkable skills, and are known for Lecture with Qigong, which can make a gym holding an audience of thousands be charged in a strong energy state. The strong External Qi energy the master radiates can not only pass through walls and heavy obstacles, but can also cross the oceans and even reach outer space. It is often heard that some Qigong masters, after many years of practice (some only practice for a short time), can penetrate the skeleton and viscera of others with their eyes and treat patients with radiation of energy from their bodies, etc.

We should take care to distinguish two aspects of this complicated situation. First, there are a few quacks who deceitfully claim that they possess "special function" and cheat people out of money and do harm to them in the name of teaching Qigong or treating patients with radiation of Qigong. These people and this sort of behavior should be exposed and then abolished. Second, some hold incorrect views concerning practicing Qigong. They believe in "special function" because some are extremely superstitious. Some are deceived by quacks and accept phenomena caused by deviation of Qigong as true ability or possession by spirits. We should strive to promote true knowledge of science and teach the correct methods of conducting and practice of Qigong.

We have encountered and treated many patients and dealt with fifty-one types of Qigong styles in the professional field. Among them, some claim that they possess "special function"; e.g., one woman teacher from an elementary school who practices Yarxin's (a type of) Qigong claims that she has "penetrating vision" and "remote perception." She says she has seen other people's internal organs and locates disease when she meets people. She forcefully radiates energy and treats the diseases of others. One nurse from a kindergarten, who practices Zhang Xiangyu's "Nature-centered Qigong," claims that she can not only diagnose and treat diseases, but can also see through the conduction of "messages" other people's "original form" before coming into the world. Do they possess "special function" according to the reported events? The answer is negative. Their so-called special function is merely hallucination, as shown by our tests and diagnosis. We have evidence for such a conclusion; e.g., the woman teacher who claimed she can penetrate a human body has conducted "penetration" on us. She says there is an upward hole in one doctor's intestines and a black cat behind another doctor's heart. That sounds incredible, but she claims she possesses a super-potency of energy for diagnosis and has been treating disease for the public for seven months. As far as being able to see one's "original form" before coming into the world is concerned, this story will collapse of itself. We have strong evidence to support our contention that they would return to a normal state when mental symptoms disappear after medical treatment. The "special function" disappeared and afterward even the patients had to admit that what they had previously seen was a hallucination.

Hallucination is a subjective experience; a sensation is perceived without corresponding stimulation of the sense organs. Since no entity exists in hallucination, it is an unreal perception and a mental derangement symptom. However, under some circumstances, normal people may occasionally have hallucinations; e.g., a person may hear someone calling their name when he is longing to see his relatives. This is the outcome of being highly focused. Likewise, normal people hearing strange sounds and seeing strange images while practicing Qigong are experiencing kinds of hallucinations but not "special function." The difference between hallucination occurring in normal people and that with deviation is that the hallucination in the latter does not disappear and the people with the deviation are in an excited and agitated state.

Why Does Ultra-deviation Occur?

What circumstances are likely to produce ultra-deviation?

1. Choosing unsuitable styles of Qigong to practice

Though most styles of Qigong have functions of curing disease and strengthening the body, it is advisable to choose the proper approach to practice according to one's physical condition or disease. An improper selection may result in a disastrous outcome. The styles associated with strong superstition are suitable for no one. They are dross mingled with Qigong and should be eliminated. In credulous people, it may produce ultra-deviation and most likely cause mental disorder; e.g., "nature-centered Qigong" and "natural Buddhist Qigong" belong to this category. They instill many primitive ideas when teaching students and the constant stimulation of these type of signals may cause fear, and subsequently cause people to become obsessed.

2. Improper methods of practice

Some people overstress concentration—inflexible ideas in the process of practicing Qigong. They misinterpret hallucination as "instinctive potency" and when this occurs, assiduously step up their practice. This situation will most likely result in ultra-deviation.

3. Improper length of time of practice

It is common sense in the field of Qigong and medical science that the time of daily practice should not be overextended. Especially for static Qigong, it is normally practiced by taking deep breaths and gradually entering a calm, static state. Being static for a long time may cause a large portion of the cerebral cortex to be restrained, and certain portions may become overexcited. This may easily cause dysfunction of the cerebral cortex, and mental symptoms will appear. Furthermore, since the practitioner's consciousness is in a trancelike state after being static for a long time, the trainee may be startled and suffer mental disorder if he hears some unexpected sounds or sees some dreadful images.

Some concerns regarding the trainees themselves

1. Diathesis

Diathesis means the trainees' disposition, medical history, and whether they are in a transitional period of their life such as menopause. If the trainees' mental background is unsound, e.g., those who have obvious antisocial and eccentric disposition, the very fastidious or narrow-minded, those extremely worried about their health, those likely to fuss over trifling matters, and those who are oversensitive and may easily accept other's or their own suggestion, improper practice may cause mental disorder. Those who have suffered from mental disease or have close relatives who have suffered from such disease are not suited to practice Qigong. If they do, it may easily induce this type of disease. Those who are in menopause or other transitional times of life are very prone to ultra-deviation.

2. Sociopsychological factors

Sociopsychological factors have great influence on one's mental state. Family background, working conditions, social position, and beliefs about life or religion are main considerations. A family member's death, failed or unfriendly relationships, divorce in the family background, disappointment, unemployment, punishment, tense relations with associates in the workplace, natural disasters, accidents, and environmental pollution have a strong impact on people. If trainees are not careful, stress may cause mental disorder. Ultra-deviation is more likely to occur in people who believe in religion or superstition and take the existence of spirits and ghosts as reality in addition to taking a superstitious approach to the practice of Qigong.

What we have discussed above implies that ultra-deviation will occur under those conditions among those who try to practice Qigong, but this is not absolutely the case. "Everything will stand with anticipation and fall without it." It would be beneficial to have a general understanding about the above-mentioned situations and realize how things can develop and hence pay close attention before beginning or in the initial period of practicing Qigong.

Preliminary study on the mechanism of ultra-deviation

There are two different points of view concerning the mechanism which causes ultra-deviation. The difference is whether one admits the existence of "energy" and the effect of "external Qigong."

Disruption of the biological field is the cause of disease.

This view admits the existence of "intrinsic energy" (Inner Qi) and "extrinsic energy" (External Qi), and believes ultra-deviation is related to the conduction, radiation, and circulation of energy. According to this viewpoint, due to the effect of "Qigong," improper practice will intensify the physical biological field of the human body (which includes sound, light, electric, magnetic, and heat waves) and cause various biological changes; may stimulate a series of changes in psychology, physiology, and biochemistry; and lead to the occurrence of mental symptoms. Tests on the effects of "intrinsic energy" and "extrinsic energy" have so far not been widely acknowledged at home or abroad as valid. Many scientists question the experimental approach of the tests, and are of the opinion they lack stability, cannot be duplicated, and were not conducted following strict scientific procedures. Therefore, this view is lacking scientific foundation.

Suggestion is the cause of disease.

This view denies the existence of "intrinsic energy" and "extrinsic energy" and implies that suggestion is the main cause of mental symptoms under special conditions. Qigong is a type of training which affects physiological functions by psychological adjustment using self-suggestion as its core. A special potent state called "Qigong state" may be reached through suggestion when practicing Qigong. This is not different from the special state induced by yoga, deep meditation, and hypnosis. In this state, most portions of the cerebral cortex are controlled and a partial portion is alert. The pons is in a remarkable state of susceptibility to change, whereas spinal nerves are partially in a state of restraint and partially in a state of change. This situation of the central nervous system can explain some phenomena which occur when practicing Qigong, e.g., "static cerebrum," "dynamic viscera," "self-initiating movement," "super muscle force," etc.

The following explanation concerning the mechanism of mental disease caused by Qigong can be made on the basis of the above: The processes of sensation, thinking, emotion, and behavior of human beings are affected by suggestion. Excessive and unhealthy suggestion under the state of Qigong may be an important reason for developing mental disease.

"Sense of energy" is an abnormal sensation caused by concentrating on certain parts of the body through conditioned reflex (I. P. Pavlov thought that suggestion is a typical conditioned reflex) under the influence of suggestion of a Qigong master and oneself. Those who are easily affected by suggestion may experience a "sense of energy," and those who are hardly affected by other's suggestion may also experience such abnormal phenomenon through constant self-suggestion. Those who are highly sensitive to suggestion may immediately perceive the existence of a "sense of energy" after they are taught Qigong or read books on Qigong. Other mental symptoms such as hallucinations and delusions have something to do with suggestion. Under the special state of Qigong, the Qigong master instills primitive and superstitious ideas into the minds of students using language, gestures, behavior, visual cues, facial expression, or through books, newspapers, and pictures. The trainees will seek the occurrence of special function (instinctive potency) such as special visual ability and special audio ability. Under these conditions, things will happen. We believe, based on comprehensive analysis of data, one will see simple light spots or rays when signals produced through other's or self-suggestion stimulate Bulaodeman 17 region of the cerebral cortex which controls the sense of vision. If the eighteenth region is stimulated, the pattern of light spots and rays will become more complicated. If the nineteenth region is stimulated, one can perceive specific images like human figures, objects, and fantasy beings. If the signals stimulate Bulouderman 41 and 42 regions of the cerebral cortex, which directs the sense of hearing, one can hear sound. According to I. P. Pavlov's theory, hallucination and wild thoughts are the outcome of different portions of the cerebral cortex producing inertial signals in the exalted range (overstimulation). The exalted signal range will predominate because of constant stimulation, and the perceptual experience and pathological phenomenon of illusory hallucination and delusion will happen spontaneously.

In addition, it has been reported that practicing Qigong may increase enkephalin in human beings, according to studies done at some institutions in China. As far as we know, psychological therapy and hypnotism may cause identical results. A hypothesis about mental disease has been raised based on data received from overseas: excessive enkephalin may be a physiological mechanism in some mental diseases. Based on this information, we may infer that deviation of Qigong may be related to mental conditions associated with increased enkephalin.

Must the Trainee "Break through the Barrier" of Deviation?

The purpose of practicing Qigong is to strengthen the body, but not all people are suited to practice Qigong. According to the opinions of some Qigong masters and relevant books, one should stop practicing Qigong whenever ultra-deviation occurs. However, some publications which proclaim the Qigong of gods and spirits stress just the opposite, e.g., *The Soul of Nature* is a book on Qigong which flatters Ms. Zhang Xiangyu. It postulates the view that "practicing Qigong is like breaking through a physical barrier, and everything will be settled after one breaks through." Actually, this is an extremely erroneous idea. The opinion of some who claim one must break through the barrier of deviation is even more absurd. To let the trainees try to break through some barrier when strong reactions or even dangerous symptoms occur is equivalent to allowing them to slip into the abyss of ultra-deviation.

It is natural to have some reactions when practicing Qigong, they may develop into deviation if one does not follow correct guidance, denies one is having a reaction, or accepts improper guidance. Qualitative changes may occur in the trainee's mental condition; deviation and reaction to Qigong occur when we neglect such changes. Those superstitious styles of Qigong practice, in which they instill various absurd ideas when teaching students; e.g., one can radiate Qigong to treat disease after one has practiced for a hundred days; one can possess "special visual ability," "special audio ability," "special ability of communication," "special ability of touch," when one enters the advanced "state of Qigong; one can talk with Buddha; one will possess three magic weapons—a sword for fighting possessive creatures and a calabash and a fan for vanquishing demons, etc.

In order to pursue these potent "special functions" some trainees become too absorbed in practice to remember food and sleep and neglect to be wary of reactions and symptoms. They think that they have entered "the advanced state of Qigong," and will cultivate "positive results" after they break through this barrier. Some patients receiving medical treatment in hospital were even convinced to try to break through the barrier. In the end, they neither broke through the "barrier" nor cultivated "positive results," but on the contrary, suffered the disastrous effects of ultra-deviation.

We can conclude that breaking through some physical or mental barrier is unrealistic and one should practice Qigong in terms of the following principles:

While learning and practicing Qigong, one should let one's instructor have a full understanding of one's living conditions, mental condition, and the development during practice (including reactions to practicing Qigong). After the occurrence of some abnormal sensations or phenomena, one should promptly confer with qualified instructors or consult relevant institutions related to psychological and psychiatric health in order to understand such phenomena. One should never handle the matter oneself and proceed blindly.

One Should Prevent Deviation When Practicing Qigong

Preventing deviation is a most important matter for people practicing Qigong. I would like to present some opinions for your reference.

Have a psychological consultation before practicing Qigong.

It is better to consult with institutions of psychological and mental health concerning one's personal condition to determine if it is proper to practice Qigong and take preventive measures if necessary. The following types of people are not fit for practice in terms of our clinical experience.

(1) Those who have suffered from symptoms of mental disease or have a member of the family suffering from such disease. Based on case-study observations, those who have suffered from various mental diseases are not suitable for practice even though they have fully recuperated. It may induce a recurrence or worsen their previous disease. A family history of mental disease means their family has had mental patients among their parents, either systems of cousins in three generations. In terms of our preliminary clinical statistics, about one-third of patients among cases of deviation have a family history of positive mental disease.

(2) Those with unsound personalities. Based on recent case observations, we find deviation of Qigong is related to personal disposition. It is suggested that the following types of people not practice it. Those who are unsociable and eccentric, sensitive and skeptical, think without logic, and are full of illusion or obsessed with certain thoughts. Moreover, those with a strong sense of suggestion may easily induce deviation since they will accept other's opinion without analysis, and be credulous about another's words. The language gestures, expression of the Qigong master or books and pictures concerning mysterious styles of Qigong may also play a great role in suggestion. Those who are extremely concerned about their situation and their health will feel discomfort and suspect they have contracted an incurable disease if they experience a "sense of energy" during practice. This concern may subsequently cause mental symptoms.

(3) Those who believe in superstition. Those who are normally superstitious and are overly religious, who believe in gods and spirits, may be susceptible to deviation according to our clinical cases. Therefore, we

think that those who are very superstitious should be extremely careful when selecting Qigong styles.

Have a clear goal for practice.

Practicing Qigong is for preventing disease and for body-strengthening. People should neither believe in superstition nor should they exclusively seek the "advanced state of Qigong" and "instinctive potency" (special function). We have had a lot of disastrous lessons in this respect; e.g., some want to possess perceptual ability through the practice of Qigong and they concentrate on this practice day and night. They even think they have obtained "special visual ability" or "special ability of communication" when mental symptoms occur and can talk daily with gods of heaven, nature, trees, etc. and eventually lose contact with the normal world and need care even in simple household activities.

The time of daily practice should not be overextended.

Though practicing up to three hours a day is accepted in the field of Qigong, being addicted to inner reflection in meditation for three consecutive hours may cause emotional disturbance and hallucinations in light of some overseas materials. In our clinical practices, we have seen lots of patients suffering from deviation who practice less than three hours a day. This may be due to many factors. But generally speaking, overextended practice time is not recommended.

Do not fear disease and abstain from medical care when deviation occurs.

One must see a doctor when mental symptoms caused by deviation occurs, especially when massive and sustained hallucinations, thought disturbance, and eccentric behavior occurs. Do not be afraid of the disease and abstain from medical treatment, instead allowing a Qigong master to try to correct the deviation. You may risk not acting in time to cure the disease.

The instructor should be responsible for his students.

We raise several suggestions on the basis of our working experience.

(1) The Qigong master should teach Qigong using a scientific approach and point out to his students that the purpose of practice is to cure disease and to strengthen the body. He should not deify Qigong and exaggerate its effects, but teach the students to practice in an easy but natural way and not to seek so-called instinctive potency, special visual ability, special audio ability, and extend their practice time.

(2) When opening training classes of Qigong, the instructor should strictly select the participants and should not accept everyone since some are not suitable for such practice. We must treat this matter seriously to avoid deviation.

(3) One should stop practicing immediately whenever hallucination and/or eccentric thought and behavior occur. The attitude of breaking through a barrier is not at all encouraged. Though some trainees have reactions like hallucination during their initial training period and continue without permanent harm, we do not think it necessary to risk such a venture.

(4) Adopt a correct attitude toward patients with deviation. We should persuade them to go to a mental hospital for professional help and encourage them to receive medicinal therapy when the deviation cannot be corrected effectively by the instructor himself.